Evidence-Based Interventions for Social Work in Health Care

Social work practice in health care requires that practitioners be prepared to meet the interdisciplinary and managed care demands for best practices in efficacious, time-limited, and culturally competent interventions, with populations across the lifespan. This text is designed to meet that demand for evidence-based practice.

The result of extensive systematic reviews, *Evidence-Based Interventions for Social Work in Health Care* provides substantive in-depth knowledge of empirically based interventions specifically for major and emerging medical diseases and health conditions particularly affecting diverse, at-risk, and marginalized populations. It outlines best practices for the psychosocial problems associated with the emerging chronic and major health conditions of the twenty-first century, such as pediatric asthma, Type 1 and Type 2 diabetes, obesity, pediatric cancer, and adult hypertension. The interventions discussed are detailed in terms of for whom, by whom, when, under what circumstances, for what duration, and for what level client system the intervention has proven most effective.

This invaluable text is suitable for students and will be a useful reference for practitioners specializing in social work in health settings.

Marcia Egan is an Associate Professor at the College of Social Work, University of Tennessee, USA.

Evidence-Based Interventions for Social Work in Health Care

Marcia Egan

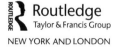

Routledge
Taylor & Francis Group

NEW YORK AND LONDON

First published 2010
by Routledge
2 Park Square, Milton Park, Abingdon, Oxon OX14 4RN

Simultaneously published in the USA and Canada
by Routledge
711 Third Avenue Avenue, New York, NY 10017

Routledge is an imprint of the Taylor & Francis Group, an informa business

Typeset in Sabon by Keyword Group Ltd

Library of Congress Cataloging-in-Publication Data
Egan, Marcia.
Evidence-based interventions for social work in health care / Marcia
Egan.
p. ; cm.
Includes bibliographical references.
1. Medical social work. 2. Chronic diseases–Social aspects.
3. Cancer in chilren–Social aspects. I. Title.
[DNLM: 1. Social Work–methods. 2. Delivery of Health Care,
Integrated. 3. Evidence-Based Practice–methods. 4. Patient Care Team.
5. Patients–psychology. W 322 E28e 2010]
HV687.E33 2010
362.2'0425–dc22   2009021812

ISBN 10: 0-7890-3559-6 (hbk)
ISBN 10: 0-7890-3560-X (pbk)
ISBN 10: 0-203-86505-7 (ebk)

ISBN 13: 978-0-7890-3559-2 (hbk)
ISBN 13: 978-0-7890-3560-8 (pbk)
ISBN 13: 978-0-203-86505-7 (ebk)

This text would not have happened were it not for two enduring aspects of my own personal and professional process. My "own true north" consistently endorses my work and my learning as evidenced in his own perseverance through many challenges and in living. Thank you, Todd. The enthusiasm and commitment of my graduate social work students inspired this text in the hope that it may help them fulfill their goal of providing their future clients with the best available practices.

Contents

Introduction

The motivation for this text arose partially from the voices in the literature calling for the use of evidence-based interventions in social work. In health care, especially, the need for practitioners skilled in interventions is supported by the transdisciplinary nature of this practice. The way we practice in health care requires that we are credible in the eyes of other health care professionals, including physicians, nurses, and psychologists.

Mullen (2008) identifies the divide between what research shows and what is actually used in practice, echoing others over the last decade. Zlotnick and Galambos (2004) note the need for workers in health care to translate evidence from other health care professions in order to delineate the interventions that best fit our clients such and indicates the relevance of systematic reviews in that endeavor. McNeill (2006) suggested that the development of evidence is one challenge, and the implementation of that which already has evidence is another. In terms of the former, limited research skills might deter development. Using interventions that have demonstrated effectiveness can be blocked when the practitioners do not have access to those interventions and/or the search skills needed to locate them. It could be assumed that practitioners have easy access to computerized databases, or reports of such interventions. However, as McNeill (2006), for one, indicates agencies may not have the resources for access and/or be reluctant to have practitioners use time to search for the evidence. The present text seeks to provide a readily available source on health care interventions with promise of efficacy. For clarity, interventions that have some support of being effective might be referred to as promising, efficacious, effective, evidence-based, or best practice. These terms are used interchangeably in the text to connote its underlying principle—that what we are after is the best currently available practices for clients in health care practice (Gambrill, 2006).

The text is based on systematic reviews on the five health disorders and diseases that are the focal points of the text. These foci were chosen because the diseases/conditions disproportionately affect diverse and vulnerable populations, most of which have prevalence and incidence rates of epic proportions. (Details of each search are provided in the Appendix.) Of course, any systematic search is limited by any unknown limitations of the databases, the English language only limit in the current search, and that intervention evaluations could exist in sources not included in the databases.

The text has a consistent structure throughout the chapters. Each chapter begins with the prevalence or incidence rates of each disorder, discussion of the nature of the disease or condition and risk factors, followed by medical treatment and regimen, the psychosocial stressors of the condition for those who have the illness and their families, and the delineation of the interventions located through the systematic review process. Each chapter concludes with the implications for practice and future research, a client scenario and questions for reflection and discussion, and a glossary of relevant terms. Lastly, the tables detailing the specifics of each intervention for each chapter are included in the relevant chapter.

The text begins with asthma in childhood and adolescence, an illness now reaching epidemic proportions, especially among minority and urban dwelling children and teens. The extent of promising interventions for pediatric asthma is heartening and may result from the lengthy extent of the research on this disease.

The second chapter is on diabetes for those with Type 1 (children and adolescents primarily), and Type 2 (primarily adults). Diabetes' prevalence rates are particularly disturbing given the scope of its negative sequelae and co-morbidities. Notably the number of interventions located for this disease is laudable, particularly those interventions substantiated with diverse client populations.

The third chapter discusses hypertension; estimates now suggest that one of every four Americans has hypertension with expectations that this ratio will only increase and do so rapidly. Hypertension affects African Americans very disproportionately.

The fourth chapter is on a topic that is gaining public and media attention: obesity. The World Health Organization now identifies obesity and being overweight as a major global health concern, one that is gaining in prevalence, and is overwhelmingly more prevalent among racially diverse populations.

The final chapter addresses an area of health care that because of its life-threatening nature and rapidly increasing rates of survival is noteworthy. This area is pediatric cancer. The number of psychosocial interventions for best practice with children and teens with cancer is at present somewhat limited. However, the literature on pediatric cancer clearly demonstrates the necessity for efficacious psychosocial interventions throughout the diagnostic and treatment phases, but just as importantly for survivors as several types of cancer now have survival rates of 90 percent or more. Social workers will have clients who at some point in their lives had pediatric cancer. Understanding the challenges faced in each phase, and the interventions with supportive evidence are crucial. Finally, the book concludes with an Appendix which details each systematic search, and references.

1 Asthma in Childhood and Adolescence

- ♦ Who is affected by pediatric asthma?
- ♦ What is asthma? What are asthma medical regimens and treatments? What are the associated family and child psychosocial stressors?
- ♦ What interventions are promising for social work implementation?
  - • Family-focused interventions
  - • Child- and adolescent-focused interventions
- ♦ Glossary
- ♦ Scenario

Introduction

Pediatric asthma receives a great deal of attention in the research literature, possibly due to its epidemic-size prevalence, and as likely to the life threatening nature of the illness. Practitioners in a variety of settings are likely to have children and families contending with the psychosocial aspects of the illness. This chapter seeks to provide the best practices for intervening with asthmatic children and youth, and with their families. For practitioners to implement these promising interventions, however, they must understand the prevalence and the nature of the disease itself. Thus, this chapter first discusses the prevalence of pediatric asthma and characteristics of the affected population, the nature of the illness, medical regimens and treatments, and the stressors on asthmatic children and their families. Following this background, the details of the 22 studies identified in the systematic review that met the criteria of the study are explicated. The chapter concludes with an exploration of the implications for practice, and future research, a glossary of relevant terms, and a scenario for discussion.

Who is Affected by Pediatric Asthma?

Asthma is the most common chronic disease among children in the U.S. (Akinbami, 2006; American Lung Association, 2007). The Centers for Disease Control & Prevention (2006b) reported that over 9 percent (i.e., 9.4 percent), or nearly seven million children in the U.S. have a diagnosis of asthma (Akinbami, 2006; Centers for Disease Control & Prevention, 2006b). The financial direct cost for one year of health care alone for pediatric asthma is nearly 15 billion dollars annually (i.e., 14.7); medications for pediatric asthma total just over an additional six billion dollars (American Lung Association, 2007). These financial costs relate to the pattern of pediatric asthma itself, including ongoing and recurrent symptoms requiring care, and acute episodes requiring recurrent emergency department visits and hospitalizations, both characteristic of a chronic illness.

The extent of the impact of pediatric asthma cannot be over-stated. Pediatric asthma is a major reason for children's use of acute medical care, including being the third leading cause of hospitalizations in those less than 15 years of age (American Lung Association, 2007). In 2004, nearly 200,000 hospitalizations, representing about three percent of all hospitalizations among children, and over three quarters of a million visits to emergency departments for children were due to their asthma (Akinbami, 2006; Centers for Disease Control & Prevention, 2006b). Akinbami notes that 6.5 million physician office visits and outpatient clinic visits for children in 2004 were for asthma (2006).

Behind those daunting statistics are the costs of the financial, psycho-social, and emotional sequelae of pediatric asthma for the children and their affected families. Asthma is the leading cause of school absenteeism, accounting for 14.6 million lost school days in 2002 alone (Centers for Disease Control & Prevention, 2006a; Pulcini, DeSisto, & McIntyre, 2007). Parents and caregivers miss work days due to the care needed by their asthmatic children with inestimable indirect cost, and lost wages, and the potential loss of jobs and, thereby, health care coverage due to absences from work (Lara et al., 2002).

Racial, Gender, and Economic Disparities in Asthma Prevalence

Childhood asthma is disproportionately prevalent among minority, poor and urban, and medically under-served populations in the U.S. (Akinbami, 2006; Akinbami & Schoendorf, 2002; Centers for Disease Control & Prevention, 2006a; Kaugars, Klinnert, & Bender, 2004; Lee, Parker, & DuBose, 2008; Lieu et al., 2002; Shegog, Bartholomew, Parcel, Sockrider, Masse, & Abramson, 2001). The statistics evidencing these disparities is striking. Not only are prevalence rates disparate for African American children, but also emergency department visits for asthma health care by black children is 200 percent and hospitalizations 250 percent higher compared to non-Hispanic white children (Akinbami, 2006).

The overall mortality (death) rate for children with asthma (just under 3 per million) continues to increase with consistently higher rates for boys in comparison to girls, and among African American children compared to their white, non-Hispanic white cohorts (Akinbami & Schoendorf, 2002). Most dramatically, the rate of death from asthma for black children is 500 percent higher than for white children with asthma (Akinbami, 2006).

Children from economically poor families and those in urban areas are more likely to have a diagnosis of asthma than are children from non-poor, and/or non-urban families (e.g., Akinbami & Schoendorf, 2002; Kaugars et al., 2004). Given the health care system Americans are currently enduring, it is not surprising that low-income children are treated more often in episodic care through emergency or urgent care centers, than in more preventive ongoing care (Fox, Porter, Lob, Holloman, Rocha, & Adelson, 2007). This limitation in medical care use is associated with inconsistent or inadequate maintenance of medical regimens, which often lead to increased acute episodes and the associated overuse of emergency medications without medical supervision (Fox et al., 2007).

Risk Factors for Pediatric Asthma

The medical causalities of asthma are extensively studied. And, though the exact cause or causal linkages for asthma are not yet known, research on possible links consistently evidences that:

- minority group membership,
- gender,
- and poverty,

are risk factors for developing asthma in childhood (e.g., Brown, Bakeman, Celano, Demi, Kobrynski, & Wilson, 2002). In combination, these factors are believed to interact with factors limiting access to ongoing, preventive medical care (e.g., being uninsured, under-insured and/or lacking funds to cover care and medications), resulting in the higher prevalence rates of asthma among minority children, and/or their greater use of emergency health care for asthma attacks (Akinbami & Schoendorf, 2002; Lieu et al., 2002; Pulcini et al., 2007).

What is Asthma?

Asthma is a chronic inflammatory disease of the airways (bronchial tubes). The inflammatory process causes re-current bronchospasms and increased mucus production resulting in difficulty in breathing with episodes of wheezing, shortness of breath, general chest tightness, and/or coughing, the latter occurring particularly at night or early morning (Centers for Disease Control & Prevention, 2005b; Sales, Fivush, & Teague, 2008). Acute episodes of asthma are life-threatening (Akinbami, 2006).

The difficulty in breathing results from hyper-sensitivity or hyper-responsivity of the airways to asthma "triggers," such as:

- dust,
- mites and insect dust,
- mold,
- chemicals,
- pollen,
- viral infections (e.g., common cold),
- and/or psychosocial or emotional stress.

Unfortunately, though the prevalence rates of childhood asthma have steadily risen since 1980, with resultant increased attention in medical research, the exact cause(s) of asthma remain largely unclear. Some authors (e.g., Burke, 2003; Kaugars et al., 2004; McCunney, 2005) suggest, however, that the cause of the disease is likely to be a combination or interaction of the following factors:

- genetic predisposition factors,
- environmental triggers,
- physical and psychosocial factors.

The most notable psychosocial factor is stress on the child, on the family, and/or in the interaction(s) of the child and her/his family (Sales et al., 2008; Sawyer, Spurrier, Whaites, Kennedy, Martin, & Baghurst, 2001; Wood et al., 2007). These physical and emotional stressors can also cause and/or contribute to acute episodes that can be life threatening (American Lung Association, 2007).

What is the Medical Treatment and Regimen for Pediatric Asthma?

The daily medical regimen for pediatric asthma includes vigilance for environmental triggers (dust, chemicals, etc.) and allergens (foods, animals, molds, etc.), and careful maintenance of medications. Consistent monitoring of the child's school classroom, playground, and recreational activities for potential environmental triggers, and routine and emergency medications are necessary. When acute symptoms appear, caregivers/parents must administer emergency medications to relieve restricted breathing and wheezing, and follow up to assure that the medications relieve the acute symptoms. In general, emergency medications are delivered in the form of an inhalant, a vaporized form of medication that is inhaled by the asthmatic. In the event that these medications do not relieve the symptoms, emergency medical care must be obtained from physicians and/or emergency rooms. In sum, the regimen for care is a 24 hour, seven day a week routine where inadvertently missed, or a lack of needed medications can result in life-threatening attacks, attacks that are often rapid in their progression from acute to critical.

Stressors on the Child

Childhood asthma has multiple, complex, and extensive effects on the child with asthma and on their family/caretakers (Ng, Li, Lou, Tso, Wan, & Chan, 2008; Wade, 2000; Weil, Wade, Bauman, Lynn, Mitchell, & Lavigne, 1999). The child with asthma experiences stress from the symptoms of the disease itself, and from acute episodes, as well as from the extensive daily medical regimens required to manage the disease.

In addition to coping with directly illness-related stressors, lifestyle adaptation to the requirements of daily medications and regimens can deter the child's achieving, and/or the timeliness of achieving their regular developmental tasks (Marsac, Funk, & Nelson, 2006; Wamboldt & Levin, 1995). Kaugars and co-authors (2004) discuss at length the complexities of asthma care and the scope of the impact of the disease on children's lives. They note in particular the research suggesting that an early onset of asthma puts asthmatic children at greater than average risk for behavior problems, and may limit their range of coping strategies. Specifically, these research findings imply that asthmatic children, particularly early-onset (younger) children, internalize more than non-asthmatic children do, and have higher rates of anxiety disorders, most notably among children experiencing more acute attacks and hospitalizations (e.g., McQuaid, Kopel, & Nassau, 2001). In brief, the psycho-emotional climate of the family is seen as pivotal in the effective management of pediatric asthma. This latter issue further endorses the importance of effective interventions by social workers.

Family Stressors and Tasks

While the child's stressors directly affect her/his emotional wellness, and may actually prompt acute attacks, the child's stress also influences the emotional well-being of his/her caretakers. The result is a reciprocal cycle in the family (child<>family/parents <>child) that can have major bearing on disease outcomes, such as exacerbations of symptoms or attacks, the frequency of emergency room visits, and/or hospitalizations (Ng et al., 2008). The links between a family's stress in managing their child's asthma, the asthmatic child's own stress, and the child's acute episodes (attacks) are documented, as is the centrality of the family in effective asthma management (Svavarsdottir, McCubbin, & Kane, 2000; Wade, 2000; Weil et al., 1999; Wood et al., 2007). These interactive stressors set the context for the complexities of asthma in children.

These complexities result in daily multiple tasks for the family. The stress of these responsibilities is influenced by, and in turn, influences the child's overall emotional well-being. In summary, the family's psychosocial stressors are related to:

- required vigilance for the presence, and elimination of environmental triggers,
- effective management of asthma symptoms,
- maintenance of medication regimens,
- prevention of asthma attacks and acute episodes.

In sum, families' tasks in their children's daily lives include ongoing coordination with school personnel concerning symptoms, medications, school and playground environmental triggers and with health care providers regarding symptoms, reactions to medications, and attacks (e.g., Kaugars et al., 2004; Parker-Oliver, 2005; Shegog et al., 2001; Wade, 2000).

Coupled with the asthma-related tasks and stressors is the ongoing parental responsibility for nurturing their child's attainment of normative developmental and the psychosocial tasks and attendant needs of their children (Parker-Oliver, 2005; Svavarsdottir et al., 2000). It was suggested early on in the literature that a family's abilities to handle these tasks is related to whether and to what extent they have a social support system in place, and whether these supports provide buffers to the stressors (Mailick, Holden, & Walther, 1994; Tal, Gil-Spielberg, Antonovsky, Tal, & Moaz, 1990; Weil et al., 1999). More recently, Horner (2004) notes that supportive networks may be needed particularly for poorer families that have less access to formal support and health services. Others report that the families of asthmatic children are overwhelmed with the multiple tasks and daily burdens and associated strain of caretaking their children (Warschburger, Von Scherin, Buchholz, & Peterman, 2002).

The factors most consistently indicated as related to effective management of the illness are the parents' coping capacities and strategies, asthma knowledge, and social support networks. Sales et al., (2008) empirically linked parental coping strategies to the quality of life of their asthmatic children. That is, mothers who use active coping strategies, rather than avoidance strategies, are more likely to manage their child's asthma well, with fewer acute episodes (Halterman, Borrelli, Fisher, Szilagyi, & Yoos, 2008; Marsac et al., 2006). Kaugars and colleagues (2004) stress the findings that parental depression, anxiety, and family conflict are strongly related to greater numbers and to the severity of acute attacks, and numbers of hospitalizations of their children. Klinnert and colleagues (2008) suggest similarly that the emotional climate in the family, in particular a negative environment, were associated with asthma severity, behavioral, and adjustment problems in their correlational study of asthmatic four year olds and their families (Klinnert, Kaugars, Strand,

& Veira, 2008). Kaugars and co-authors (2004) suggest that family environments characterized by conflict, aggressive behaviors, and a lack of nurturing may place some children at a higher risk of having asthma, and poorer outcomes for asthmatic children in such families, than children in families without those characteristics. The risk factors in combination characterize the lives of many children, perhaps those most vulnerable to many psychosocial and environmental risks.

Obviously, the directionality of these relationships and contexts require much further empirical study. However, it also seems that interventions which are empowering, focus on asthma management skills, target reducing stress and anxiety, and/or are supportive of parent caregivers are appropriate.

Promising Interventions for Practice

The 22 studies located in the systematic review that met the criteria of this systematic review are discussed below. First, the 11 family-centered interventions are discussed, followed by discussions of the 11 child-centered intervention evaluations located in the present research.

Family and Parent Centered Interventions

Though not at all surprising, given the affirmation that the family is pivotal in effective management of asthma in children, much of the empirical literature offering promising interventions in pediatric asthma focus on family-centered interventions. The evidence-based family-centered interventions located through the systematic review utilized several modes of delivery. Overall, these interventions included modalities as follows:

- multi-family group,
- educational,
- problem solving,
- parent-only small group,
- individual family therapy.

Some studies included multiple modalities in one intervention package (e.g., Bonner, Zimmerman, Evans,Trigoyen, Resnick, & Mellins, 2002; McCarthy, Herbert, Brimacombe, Hansen, Wong, & Zehman, 2002).

Multi-Family Group Interventions

Overall, 11 family-centered interventions in pediatric asthma were located. Of these, five studies implemented and evaluated a multi-family group (MFG) intervention either as the sole modality, or in combination with other modalities. Three of the five studies evaluating MFG found were randomized control group designs—the "gold standard"—of evaluative clinical research (Bonner et al., 2002; LaRoche, Koinis-Mitchell, & Gualdron, 2006; Walders, Keresma, Schluchter, Redline, Kirchner, & Drotar, 2006). The effectiveness suggested for the MFG approach in this area is promising as the multi-family group intervention is also reported as effective regarding depression and anorexia nervosa among family members (e.g., Honig, 2005; Lemmens, Eisler, Migerode, Heireman, & Demyttenaere, 2007). By way of reference, the reader is reminded that a multi-family group intervention combines parents/caretakers and their children of several families into one group for treatment.

The Bonner et al. (2002) RCT study speaks to the racial disparity in pediatric asthma prevalence rates. The sample was ethnically diverse with African American (25 percent) and Latino (75 percent) families in two clinics in a university hospital. A bi-lingual family coordinator conducted all interventions in the clinics. The control group received only usual clinic care. The intervention group received combined interventions including several educational multi-family group (MFG) sessions, individual family supportive services, and coordinated visits for families' collaboration with their physicians. The study occurred in cohort groups of seven families each over a period of three months. Bonner and colleagues provide detailed information on each session of the educational multi-family group, on training individual families in partnering with physicians, and on preparing for each physician appointment. In addition, the treatment group families were contacted by phone by the coordinator on a weekly basis. The findings of the study demonstrated that the intervention was effective in reducing all outcome measures (e.g., asthma knowledge, medications, and self-efficacy).

A multi-family group intervention (T1) was compared to a standard psycho-educational intervention (T2) in a randomized, three-group design with minority, urban, and economically poor families and their asthmatic children by LaRoche et al. (2006). Participants randomized to the third group (control group) received only usual medical care. The MFG intervention was significantly more effective in decreasing emergency department visits, and increasing parent knowledge of asthma and asthma management skills than either the standard psycho-educational intervention or usual care. The researchers provide details of these interventions, and discuss culturally competent asthma management, both facilitating replication of the study. Though limited by small sample size, these findings are promising given the importance of the family's abilities in effectively managing their child's asthma, and the racial disparities in prevalence, mortality, and morbidity of the disease noted previously.

Walders and colleagues (2006) conducted an RCT two-group study of a multi-modal intervention combining education, a MFG intervention, and cognitive behavioral individual family problem solving interventions compared to only medical care (i.e., usual care). Participants were recruited from multiple sites, including outpatient clinics, inpatient units, and emergency departments and were racially diverse. Education was provided in a series of sessions in multi-family group format concentrating on the physiology of asthma, environmental triggers, and the proper use of medications. In addition, brief cognitive behavioral problem solving therapy was provided to individual families in the treatment group. The study included availability of 24-hour phone contact with a nurse for questions and advice for the treatment group participants. Significant results included increased quality of life for the children and reduction in emergency room use.

One study combined an MFG intervention with empowerment strategies in a matched (demographics and asthma severity) quasi-experimental two-group comparison study. The control group (n=28) implemented a traditional multi-family group educational intervention, and the intervention group (n=29) implemented a MFG intervention enhanced with empowerment interventions in primary care settings (McCarthy et al., 2002). The study utilized baseline, post-intervention, and post six-month follow up measurements. Though findings are limited by the study's small and non-randomized sample, they provide additional support for multi-family education groups particularly those incorporate empowerment interventions in increasing parents' sense of control, abilities in providing care to their children care, and in making decisions in assessing symptoms, and needed medication and medical care.

In a two-group pre-post design, Toelle and colleagues (1993) evaluated the effect of a two, 2-hour session MFG intervention on knowledge of the disease, triggers, and medications plus preparation for families' asthma management planning with their physicians. The design included the treatment group (n=65) and a control group (n=55) that received only usual medical care. Findings included significantly increased asthma knowledge and decreased number of emergency physician and emergency department visits in the treatment group.

In summary, the evidence is promising for multi-family group interventions and incorporating educational content for asthma management in MFG interventions, particularly with diverse client populations. Some studies utilized rigorous methodologies and had significant findings on outcomes. Overall, these studies can be replicated for further evidence of efficacy, and provide sufficient intervention details for implementation by practitioners in work with families of asthmatic children in a variety of settings.

Small Group Interventions with Parents/Caretakers

Three evaluations of small group interventions with parents of asthmatic children only were located in the review, two of which were randomized, control studies, and one was a quasi-experimental design.

Utilizing RCT methodology, Gebert and colleagues (1998) examined the effectiveness of a training program in small group sessions for parents only with separate groups for children plus a follow-up individual family session (T1) compared to group training only (T2) and to usual care in a randomized clinical trial in a three-group RCT design. Their findings support the effectiveness of the training with follow up individual family sessions over both training only and over usual care only. Based on the findings, Gebert and co-authors stress the importance of long-term follow-up with families and their asthmatic children.

The study by Evans et al. (1999) is notable for the purpose of this text due to its large sample size (T = 515; C = 518), RCT block design with baseline, post-intervention, and post-every two-month follow up measurements completed over the course of the two-year study, and that masters-level social workers implemented all interventions. Participants were inner city children (5–11 years old) and their caretakers/parents, recruited from pediatric and chest clinics of a university hospital; three-quarters of the children were African American and 17 percent were Hispanic. After baseline measures were completed, children were randomly assigned in blocks of six to eight children to the intervention or control groups. The intervention included two small session groups for adults (parents and caretakers) plus one individual family session after the conclusion of the group intervention; the children's small group intervention (two sessions) was implemented after the conclusion of the parent group intervention.

The research examined the efficacy of a small group intervention to teach and encourage parents and caretakers' effective communication with their physicians, control of environmental triggers and asthma education; in addition, non-allergic pillows, and mattress covers were supplied, and needed referrals to community resources were coordinated. All group sessions for adults and for children used the *A+Asthma* curriculum on triggers and symptoms, environmental control, problem solving asthma symptoms and episodes, and, for the parents/caretakers, effective communicating with physicians. Outcome measures included health and severity indicators (e.g., symptom free days, hospitalizations), and two widely accepted psychological scales (the Brief Symptom Inventory and the Child Behavior Checklist). Findings included improved health status, reduced asthma morbidity, and improved behavior in the children as measured by the Child Behavior Checklist, and reduced use of emergency services each in the intervention group compared to the control group. This research is notable in addition to its sample size, but for its use of validated outcome measurement instruments.

With some methodological limitations, Tal and colleagues (1990) implemented a family system-based educational intervention in quasi-experimental, non-random, comparison two-group pilot study with a convenience sample of asthmatic children and their parents. The control group received usual medical care without the intervention. The small group family-system based educational intervention involved six two-hour delineated educational sessions with parents in one group and their children in a separate group. Findings were that children in the intervention group were more responsible for their own daily care and medication, and participated more often in decisions concerning their school absences compared to children in the usual care group. Second, the parents were more positive concerning the independence dynamic in their family (MOOS Family Environment Scale) after the intervention than were their respective cohorts in the control group.

In summary, small group interventions—a long held traditional intervention for social work—has some promising evidence for work with families of asthmatic children for parents and for children in separate small groups with and without the addition of single-family sessions.

Individual Family Interventions

Yorke and Shuldman (2009) summarize their systematic review of the effectiveness of family therapy on the use of asthma medications and lung volume expiration in comparison to medication alone (usual care) for the Cochrane Collaboration. Though only two studies met the inclusion criteria of the Collaboration (only RCT studies were included), the authors found that those two studies had promising results for medication use plus family therapy intervention. Unfortunately, the outcome measures of those two studies were only medication and medical outcomes and, thus, did not meet the criteria of the present systematic review. However, three studies, each of which were randomized and controlled studies, evaluating the effectiveness of family therapy with individual families of asthmatic children were located in the present systematic review that met current criteria.

Educational interventions delivered at home with individual low-income, African American families with asthmatic children were evaluated in a RCT study with pre/post-3 month and post-12 month measurements (Brown, Bakeman, et al., 2002). The program utilized the revised and pilot tested *Wee Wheezers* curriculum. Participants were recruited from specialty clinics and primary physician offices and randomly assigned to either the treatment or control groups. The educational program involved eight weekly sessions with outcome measures targeted at parental ability to monitor asthma symptoms, symptom-free days, and parental quality of life. Brown and colleagues report that families with younger children had significantly improved post-intervention scores than families with older children. The authors suggest that parents of younger children may be more highly motivated to respond to the educational program than those with older children.

Onnis et al. (2001) examined the effectiveness of family therapy (6–8 sessions) plus medication with individual families (T = 10) compared to medications alone (C = 10) with random assignment to either treatment or control groups. Findings suggest that family therapy plus medication is more effective than medication alone in decreasing the number of asthmatic attacks, improving medication use, and improving family functioning. These findings are limited by the small sample size, but lend some promise to for *value added* approach.

Ng and colleagues (2008) examined the effect of family therapy plus medication (n = 23) versus medication alone (n = 23) on the efficacy the value-added intervention on several outcome measures in a pediatric chest clinic. The measures were lung function, self-report scales on children's adjustment to asthma, and on parents' asthma efficacy in managing their child's asthma, anxiety, and emotional well-being, quality of life and well-being (SF-12 Short Form) in a randomized waitlist-controlled crossover clinical trial design. The researchers found consistently improved children's airway function, and parental asthma efficacy, physical health, and emotional well-being in the treatment group compared to the control group after intervention, and at follow up.

Overall, these studies lend support to family-centered interventions in the area of pediatric asthma as a best practice approach. Though further evidence will be a benefit, the research to date includes modalities appropriate for social work practice. This evidence, whether in MFG, small groups, or one-on-one family interventions, is augmented by the availability of substantiated curriculum on asthma. In addition, given the racial distribution of the prevalence of pediatric asthma discussed earlier in this chapter, the samples are diverse with nine of the studies including African Americans. (See Table 1.1 for summarizations of the research studies of family-centered interventions discussed above.)

Child-Centered Interventions

There is some evidence of promise from previous reviews, though constrained by criteria involved, concerning interventions targeting asthmatic children themselves. For example, Guevara and colleagues (2003) completed a systemic evaluation of RCT only studies on the effectiveness of educational interventions with children. They report that the educational interventions located were efficacious in improving lung function, self-efficacy, and reducing school absenteeism. A more recent meta-analysis of studies using randomized, control treatment designs by Coffman and colleagues (2008) found that educational interventions that compared education to usual care demonstrated statistically significant decreases in hospitalizations and emergency room visits for children with moderate asthma. However, in terms of the present discussion, those studies did not include psychosocial outcomes, nor provide sufficient detail for replicating the intervention.

Table 1.1 Family-centered interventions in childhood asthma

Author (year)	Objective	Design	Intervention	Mode	Sample	Outcome measures	Results	Notes
Bonner et al. (2002)	To evaluate intensive multi-modal intervention for urban Latino & African American families	RCT; 2-group; pre/post over 3 months; C = Usual care only	Education, problem solving counseling, phone support, conjoint family & physician appointments, environmental assessment	MFG & single family sessions + home visits	T = 50 families, C = 50 families; ~75% Latino, ~22% African American; nearly 90% on Medicaid; 4–19 y/o	Asthma knowledge self-efficacy, medication & treatment adherence, Western health belief acceptance; measures in English & Spanish	T1 = all outcome measurements improved	Small sample, only 1 post measure; unique in cultural competence approach & partnering with families at physician appointments
Brown, Bakeman et al. (2002)	To evaluate home-based asthma education program for low-income families	RCT; 2-group; pre/post, & post 3 & 12 months; C = Usual care	*Wee Wheezers at Home*; 8 sessions	Single family	T = 49 & C = 46; 89/90% African American; 80/84% low SEC; 1–8 y/o	Severity of asthma, asthma management, & Caregiver's QOL scales	T1 = ↓ asthma severity & ↑ asthma management & ↑ QOL	Significant results for families with 1–3 y/o, not families with older children

(continued)

Table 1.1 Family-centered interventions in childhood asthma *(continued)*

Author (year)	Objective	Design	Intervention	Mode	Sample	Outcome measures	Results	Notes
Evans et al. (1999)	To evaluate education + empowering program with multi-racial families & children	RCT multi-site 2-group, pre/post & post each 2 months over 2 years; blocked & children randomly assigned in blocks of 6–8 children; C=Usual care only	2 session-groups for adults & for children + individual family session; A+Asthma curriculum & effectively communicating with physicians	Small group + 1 individual family session	5–11-year-old children & their families; 75% African American & 17% Hispanic; T = 515; C = 518	Symptomatic days, Brief Symptom Inventory (BSI), CBCL	T = ↓ symptom days, improved BSI & CBCL scores	Multi-site; implemented by social workers; diverse population; clear intervention details provided; large sample
Gebert et al. (1998)	To compare training with follow-up sessions with training alone	RCT; 3 group; pre/post at 12 months; T1 = training + follow-up sessions; T2 = training only; C = Usual care only	5-day asthma knowledge & self-management education & single family sessions q months/×6	Small group with parents & children + follow-up	T1 = 27, T2 = 29, C = 25; children 7–14 y/o	Health Locus of Control Scale, asthma self-management skills, school absences	T1 = ↑ self-management skills, ↓ school absences, ↑ Internal Health Locus of Control	
LaRoche et al. (2006)	To compare MFG intervention with standard psycho-education group	RCT; 3 groups: pre-1 year & post-1 year; T1 = MFG; T2 = standard psycho-education; C = Usual care	Quasi-experimental 2-group comparison	MFG	T1 = 12, T2 = 12, C = 9; 73% Hispanic & 27% African American, all low SEC; 7–13 y/o	Parent asthma knowledge & management & ED visits	T1 = ↑ asthma knowledge, management skills & ↓ ED visits	Cultural competence emphasis in revising validated scales; clear intervention details; small sample

Study	Purpose	Design	Intervention	Type	Sample	Measures	Results	Limitations
McCarthy et al. (2002)	To compare empowerment MFG + traditional education & traditional education group	Quasi-experimental 2-group comparison; C=traditional education group; pre/post & post 6 months; groups matched on demographics & asthma severity	Multi-family empowerment group three sessions+ monthly phone contact + usual care	MFG	T1 = 29 & C = 28; children 3–16 y/o; all children newly diagnosed with asthma	Parent Sense of Control (SOC), asthma knowledge, ability to care for child & ability to make care decisions	T1 = ↑ SOC, asthma knowledge, ability to care for child & decision making ability	Small sample; non-randomized; clear intervention details; implements Dunst & Trivette model
Ng et al. (2008)	To evaluate family therapy + meds compared to meds alone	RCT waitlist cross-over 2-group design (T & C); C = Usual care (meds alone)	Systemic family therapy	Single family	T = 23; C = 23	SF-12 Short Form, Parental asthma self-efficacy scale	T = ↑ parental efficacy, improved physical health & emotional well being	Small sample
Onnis et al. (2001)	To evaluate family therapy + usual care	RCT; 2 groups; children matched (gender, age, family composition, SEC); pre/post; T = systemic family therapy + medications; C = UC only	Systemic family therapy (Milan); 6–8 sessions in 3 phases	Single family	T = 10, C = 10; 6–13 y/o, 50% male & 50% female; lower and middle SEC	# of attacks, medication use; Wyltwyck Family Task	T1 = ↓ # attacks, medication use & improved Family Task sub-scales & stress	Small sample size; Family Task measures not used in C group

(continued)

Table 1.1 Family-centered interventions in childhood asthma (*continued*)

Author (year)	Objective	Design	Intervention	Mode	Sample	Outcome measures	Results	Notes
Tal et al. (1990)	To evaluate family-systems based asthma education	Quasi-experimental 2-group comparison; convenience sample; pre/post 3 & 12 months; C=UC	Family Asthma School; six 2-hour weekly sessions	Children group & parent group	T=36, C=20 children & families; no demographics provided	MOOS Family Environment Scale	T = ↑ MOOS subscales & ↑ child's self-management	Small non-random sample; clear intervention details
Toelle et al. (1993)	To evaluate a combined intervention	Quasi-experimental, 2-group comparison; pre/post & post 3 & 6 months; C=UC	Family asthma education, two 2-hour sessions + physician, pharmacist, nurse, teacher asthma management training	MFG + asthma management training group	T=65, C=55 & families; average age 9 y/o; 58–70% male	Symptom frequency; lung function tests; asthma knowledge; ED/unscheduled physician visits	T=↑ knowledge; ↓ ED/physician visits	Small non-random sample; confound in mailing education materials to T group non-attenders
Walders et al. (2006)	To evaluate intervention for under-treated asthmatic children & families	Quasi-experimental RCT 2-group, randomized block by child age (4–9 y/o & 1–12 y/o); pre/post & post 6 & 12 months; C=UC	Combined education and cognitive behavioral problem solving therapy + education sessions + 6 follow-up sessions + 24 hr. phone nurse availability	MFG + single family	T=89, C=86 children & their families; all English speaking; 4–12 y/o; 71/73% male, 82/88% African American	Children & parents' QOL; symptom scores; ED visits	T=↓ ED visits; both T & C; ↑ QOL	Small sample size; urban tertiary hospital ED setting; clear intervention details; equivocal results

Notes: T = intervention/treatment group; T1 = 1st intervention group; T2 = 2nd intervention group; T3 = 3rd intervention group; C = control or comparison group; UC = usual care (e.g., physician visit, medication); MFG = multi-family group; ED = Emergency Department.

The studies identified in Guevara's study are included in the discussion below if they met the criteria of present systemic review concerning appropriateness for social work practitioners, sufficient detail for replication of the intervention and of the evaluative design, and included a psychosocial outcome, rather than only medical outcome measures (e.g., lung volume). Eleven studies evaluating the effectiveness of child-centered interventions were found. Of these 11, seven were implemented in schools and four were implemented in other settings.

School-Based Interventions

Notably much of the research on interventions that target asthmatic children themselves involve interventions located in schools. As suggested by Clark and co-authors (2009), while research on interventions targeting the possible causalities of asthma attacks in individual child-focused interventions may seem logical, such approaches are less efficient and more variable in implementation than programmatic interventions implemented in children's collective environments, such as schools, and health care clinics.

Accordingly, the following discussion begins with delineation of the seven studies of school-based interventions. Following this discussion, four other studies evaluating the effectiveness of individually targeted interventions implemented in other settings that offer promise found in the present research are discussed within the two categories of school-based and other settings. Within the former category, three school-based interventions that implemented the *Open Airways* curriculum are discussed first.

Early in the history of research on interventions with asthmatic children, Evans and colleagues (1987) evaluated a school-based curriculum, *Open Airways*. The 12 schools in the study were matched in pairs according to the demographics of the schools; after matching, one of each pair was randomly assigned to intervention with the other remaining six assigned as control schools. Children in the schools between eight and 11 years of age participated in the study. *Open Airways* is six one-hour sessions with small groups of eight to 12 children based on child-oriented education. The program focuses on asthma management skills, asthma self-efficacy, using medications appropriately, identifying triggers, and appropriate physical activity. The researchers report that the intervention was more effective in increasing management skills, self-efficacy, and on school performance tests in the intervention groups compared to the control group.

A more recent research study, also evaluating the *Open Airways* curriculum, in four inner city schools used a two-group, pre-/post, quasi-experimental design implemented in schools, with the intervention group receiving the curriculum—*Open Airways*—plus five monthly nurse home visits (Velsor-Friedrich, Pigott, & Louloudes, 2004). The control group received medical care only (usual care). All participants were African American children with asthma. Outcome measures included an asthma knowledge scale, an asthma self-efficacy scale, a self-esteem scale and health indicators (e.g., attacks). The findings showed significantly improved health outcomes, efficacy, knowledge, and self-esteem in the treatment group compared to the control group. However, the non-random design, and small sample size limits generalizing of the findings.

One study evaluated a program with urban, medically under-served, African American, asthmatic children (N = 243) aged six to ten years in 14 elementary schools (Levy, Heffner, Stewart, & Beeman, 2006). The evaluation involved randomization of the schools to the intervention group or to the usual care (control) group. The design, a longitudinal three-year study, implemented pre-test, post-test, and follow-up assessments after the intervention. School nurses provided education with the *Open Airways* curriculum in weekly small groups with the children, and monitored school absences, and symptoms, coordinated care services with the children and their families, and school staff and medical providers, and made at-home visits on the fifth day of the program. Outcome measurements included the children's absenteeism, emergency health care use, hospitalizations, asthma knowledge, appropriate medication use, symptom monitoring, and management skills. Each outcome measure was significantly improved in the intervention group compared to the usual care group at each post-intervention point.

Horner (2004) evaluated an intervention comprised of nine 15-minute bi-weekly sessions on self-management for third through fifth graders with participating multi-racial schools randomly assigned to intervention and control groups. Analysis of measurements at baseline, post-intervention, post-six and post 12-month points demonstrated that children in the intervention group had reduced asthma severity (i.e., symptoms and acute episodes) and school absenteeism, and increased daily management of their asthma compared with those in the control group. This study is particularly useful for practitioners as it includes very detailed descriptions of the weekly sessions.

McGhan and colleagues (2003) evaluated an asthma education program (*Roaring Adventures of Puff-RAP*) in a two-group randomized, pre-post study implemented in 18 elementary schools in Canada with seven to 13 year olds. Randomization occurred at the school level. The intervention was implemented in six one-hour interactive, age-appropriate sessions centered on asthma management skills, health status, and quality of life. Findings on health status measures (e.g., emergency doctor visits, shortness of breath, activity restrictions), and school absenteeism in the treatment group were improved compared to the control group. These findings are limited by the small sample size, and, possibly, by the prevalence of children in the study with only mild asthma, and/or by the instructors in the program, who received brief training only in the curriculum. However, replicability of the intervention is enhanced given the details of the intervention provided by the authors.

Shaw, Marshak, Dyjack, and Neish (2005) evaluated a school-based curriculum intervention on asthma knowledge, quality of life, self-efficacy, and self-management with tenth graders in a rigorously designed RCT two-group study, with delayed intervention (i.e., control group) in two high schools. The treatment and control groups were matched on socio-demographic characteristics and ethnicity. The intervention was a nine-module, two hours each on asthma physiology, triggers, and management. Measurements on the domains of interest were completed pre-intervention and at one, three and six weeks post-intervention. Self-efficacy scores significantly improved from baseline to post-test in the treatment group, but did not maintain at later measurement points.

Joseph and co-researchers (2006) evaluated a multi-media, web-based asthma management skills program (*Puff City*) compared to general referral to the web in a RCT study of high school students aged 15–19 years (grades nine through eleven) in six inner city high schools in Detroit. Students in these schools were 98 percent African American and one-half were on Medicaid. The recruitment strategy was a mailing to the student and their parents inviting them to participate in the study, including consent forms for both the parent/caretaker and student, a questionnaire on any history of asthma diagnosis, symptoms, treatment, and/or medication use in the previous 30 days. Eligible students (n = 314) from those returning the information and consent forms were randomly assigned within their school to participate in *Puff City* (n = 182) or to a control group (n = 162) that received a list of generic asthmas education websites. Randomization through a computer randomization program included school, grades level, gender and a physician diagnosed asthma condition.

The web-based program was informed by two theories: social learning and adolescent learning. The web-based program, *Puff City,* is tailored for adolescents, and developed on the asthma education guidelines of the National Asthma Education and Prevention Program, and formulated on the transtheoretical and health belief models. Central objectives of the program are to motivate behavior change in medication adherence, stopping smoking, asthma trigger avoidance offered in four interactive sessions that the students were required to complete in six months. Outcome measures occurred at baseline, and during each session after the first, including measurements of medication adherence, symptom frequency, school absences, the number of days of restricted activity, of ED visits, and of hospitalizations. Outcome findings demonstrated that the multi-media intervention was effective in improving medication adherence, reducing symptom days, absenteeism, and hospitalizations, but did not affect the frequency of ED visits or quality of life measures. The study provides promising results in reaching an otherwise described as a hard-to-reach population through multi-media technology reflective of the attraction of technology to this age group. The rigor of the recruitment, selection, and randomization processes support the promise of these findings as well.

Overall, the school-based interventions evidencing promise for intervening with asthmatic children used comparison, control, and randomized designs and often validated curricula developed for intervention in pediatric asthma. This is good news for asthmatic children and for practitioners, just as Clark, Mitchell, and Rand (2009) suggest, intervening with children in their most in-common settings affords gains in costs, and developmental age appropriateness as well. Lastly and notably, the majority of the interventions based in schools took place in urban settings with minority populations.

Interventions in Other Settings

Research evaluating interventions with asthmatic children has also been implemented outside school settings. Four studies implemented in non-school settings were located in the research that met the criteria of the study; the discussion of these studies follows. The settings of these interventions included pediatric clinic, health care, and physician office settings.

Colland (1993) employed an RCT design with two control groups, and one experimental group in an 18-month small group educational program intervening with eight to 13 year olds recruited in six pediatric clinics. Participants were matched by demographic characteristics and baseline coping with asthma and asthma severity scale scores, and then randomly assigned to one of three groups: treatment, placebo (information only in one session), and control (usual care). The program involved ten 1-hour sessions combining education for asthma self-management, role-playing, and relaxation techniques enhanced by cognitive behavior therapy. The intervention was effective in increasing coping with asthma capacities and knowledge at post-test, and at follow up (6 months post-intervention). Colland provides extensive details of the intervention program sessions, thus facilitating replication of the intervention.

Krishna and co-researchers (2006) evaluated a multi-media computer program (*IMPACT*) in clinics with children and their families while they awaited health care appointments. The treatment and control (usual care) groups in the sample were primarily white, non-Hispanic (41 percent and 45 percent, respectively), aged seven to 17 years; the parents were similarly primarily white, non-Hispanic. Those in the control group received standard care including asthma information fact sheets (e.g., triggers, medication use, prevention of symptoms, and asthma control strategies), verbal instructions, and demonstrations of techniques (e.g., inhalant use). Those children and parents in the intervention group received each of those elements of usual care plus the interactive multi-media asthma education program during their regular office visits. Analysis showed that post-tests on all measures (i.e., asthma knowledge, quality of life, health indices, health resource use, lung function) were significantly improved in those in the intervention group. Of benefit for replication is that the media program is described in detail, as are the methodological steps in the study.

Perrin and colleagues (1992) evaluated an intervention comprised of asthma education and stress management techniques for six to 14 year olds in physician offices in an RCT two-group study. The four two-hour weekly session intervention was provided to those in the waitlist control group after completion of evaluation of the treatment group. Though parents were invited to attend the educational sessions if they wished, intervention focused on the children and on child outcomes. Outcome measures were the Child Behavior Checklist (CBCL), asthma knowledge scale, stress scale, school attendance monitoring, and the daily amount of time the child was in recreational activities. Perrin and co-authors report decreased absenteeism, and improved CBCL scores on its Total Problems and Internalizing sub-scales, and on the asthma knowledge scale in the intervention group. Of particular interest are their findings that each of these sub-scale scores differed by gender at both pre- and post-test points with girls scoring higher on each at each point.

McPherson and co-authors (2006) report on an evaluation of an educational multimedia program to improve self-management skills in asthmatic children in three asthma outpatient clinics. The RCT study used a baseline, one and six month follow up design with 101 seven to 14-year-old children receiving asthma care services. Participants were randomized to the control group (receiving an asthma information booklet alone) or to the intervention group (booklet plus *The Asthma File,* a multi-media interactive CD-ROM) + home visits that included a laptop with the CD program). The *Asthma File* program may be particularly attractive to children and teens as it utilizes a video-game approach with a secret-agent theme. The program was pilot tested for one year prior to its implementation in this study; details of the program are provided. Results demonstrated that the intervention group had improved asthma knowledge, increased internal locus of control, used less oral steroid medications, and had fewer school absences than the control group.

The interventions targeting children themselves, whether in schools or in other settings, are advantageous due to their use of age-appropriate curricula, and to the rigor of their methodological designs. In sum, these interventions show promise for efficacious practice in a variety of settings, any of which are social work settings. (See Table 1.2 for summarizations of the interventions with children discussed above.)

Table 1.2 Child-centered interventions in childhood asthma

Author (year)	Objective	Design	Intervention	Mode	Sample	Outcome measures	Results	Notes
Colland (1993)	Evaluate 18-month education program	RCT; matched by demographics & baseline coping scores; pre/post & post 6 months; C1 = information only in 1 session C2 = UC	10 one-hour sessions on asthma self-management with role playing, relaxation techniques & cognitive behavior interventions	Small group	8–12.7 y/o; T = 48; C1 = 34; C2 = 30	Coping with asthma & knowledge scales	↑ Coping with asthma, & ↑ knowledge in intervention group	Details of intervention is extensive; groups matched
Evans et al. (1987)	Evaluate school-based health education program	2-group RCT matching pairs of 12 schools (T and C); baseline & follow-up	*Open Airways* in six 1-hour sessions	Small group	8–11 y/o; T = 117, C = 87; 3rd–5th graders	Asthma management skills, self-efficacy, medication use, identifying triggers, & school attendance	↑ Management skills & ↓ # & duration of attacks & ↑ school achievement scores in T group	Curriculum used is widely evaluated

	Purpose	Design	Delivery	Sample	Measures	Results	Comments
Horner (2004)	Compare education in multi-racial schools	Quasi-experimental comparison design; randomized at school level; baseline, post 6 and 12 month measures	Nine 15 minute bi-weekly sessions in schools with 5th graders	Small group	8–12 y/o; 47% African American, 23% Mexican American; T=22; C=22	Asthma severity index, school absenteeism, asthma management	↑ Asthma management & ↓ asthma severity & absenteeism	Useful details of intervention per session; limited by small sample size
Joseph et al. (2006)	Evaluate a multi-media program with teens in 6 inner city schools	RCT pre & post 12 month design; T=multi-media; C=referral to web only	*Puff City*- a multi-media, computer, 4- module program tailored to teens available for 12 months at school	Single student	15–19 year olds; 98% African American; N=314; T=182 & C=162	Medication adherence, symptom frequency, absenteeism, ED visits, & hospitalizations	↑ Adherence, & ↓ absenteeism, symptom days, ED visits & hospitalizations	Details of design provided; large sample size
Krishna et al. (2006)	Evaluate a multi-media computer program asthma education	RCT design; baseline, post 12 month measures; T=41 (UC + multi-media program); C=35 (UC)	Multi-media computer asthma education program (*IMPACT*) in clinics + UC; C (UC)	1:1 child & 1:1 parent	T=41; C=35; 41% & 45% white, non-Hispanic; 7–17 y/o	↑ Asthma knowledge & management, health resource use, health indicators, lung function	Significantly ↑ asthma knowledge, management skills scores, reduced ED use, and ↑ lung function in treatment group	Very detailed design & media program

(continued)

Table 1.2 Child-centered interventions in childhood asthma *(continued)*

Author (year)	Objective	Design	Intervention	Mode	Sample	Outcome measures	Results	Notes
Levy et al. (2006)	Evaluate 3-year program of education + coordinating resources with medically under-served teens	RCT, 2-group design; T=8 schools C=6 schools (UC); pre/post and follow up through the 3 year program	School-based education: *Open Airways*; weekly monitoring of students, coordination with children, families, providers & school personnel	Small group + 1:1 care coordination	African American 6–10 year olds in 14 elementary schools; N=243; T=115, C=128	Absenteeism, ER use, symptoms, hospitalizations, & asthma knowledge & management skills	↑ Appropriate medication use, symptom monitoring & management, ↓ absenteeism, & ED visits & hospitalizations	Widely evaluated curriculum; longitudinal design; details of analysis & limitations of design
McGhan et al. (2003)	Evaluate school-based education (*Roaring Adventures of Puff*)	2-group RCT; randomly assigned by school (N=18) pre/post design	Six 1-hour interactive age-appropriate educational sessions on asthma management skills	Small group	T=76, 82% white, C=86, 74% white; 7–13 year olds	Health status indicators (e.g., emergency visits, shortness of breath), daily activities, quality of life & school absenteeism	↓ Health status indicators ↓ ED visits, & school absences	Limited by small sample size, & possible skew in sample to children w/ mild asthma; clear details of intervention provided

Citation	Aim	Design	Intervention	Setting	Sample	Measures	Results	Comments
McPherson et al. (2006)	Evaluate a CD ROM asthma program	RCT 2-group comparison study; baseline, 1 and 6 month post design; T=information & booklet + home visit + CD; C=booklet only	CD-ROM multimedia program (*The Asthma File*) + home visits + information & booklet compared to booklet only	Single child & family	N=101; T=50; C=49	Asthma knowledge, self-management, Locus of Control, school attendance, oral medications	↑ Asthma knowledge & Internal Locus of Control; ↓ oral medication use & school absences	Useful details of the CD-ROM program; limited by the small sample size
Perrin et al. (1992)	Evaluate an asthma & stress management education program	RCT: 2-group; T=education + stress management; C=same intervention, after conclusion of the T group	Four 2-hour weekly sessions on asthma knowledge, physiology, symptoms, & triggers, exercises for relaxation & coping with children & parents	Small group	6 to 14 year olds; T=29; C=27; white (85%); middle to upper SEC (90%)	CBCL, asthma knowledge, stress, school attendance, daily recreational activities daily journals, asthma severity scale	↓ School absence & CBCL Internalizing & Total Problem sub-scales & ↑ asthma knowledge	Differences by gender; limited due to small sample size, high dropout rate; details of the intervention are provided

(continued)

Table 1.2 Child-centered interventions in childhood asthma *(continued)*

Author (year)	Objective	Design	Intervention	Mode	Sample	Outcome measures	Results	Notes
Shaw et al. (2005)	Evaluate asthma curricula based on social cognitive theory	RCT 2-group study w/ delayed intervention; pre & post tests; T=school 1; C=school 2- delayed intervention	Nine 2-hour sessions on asthma knowledge, & management	Small group	10th graders (N=122); ¾ female; included asthmatic & non-asthmatic children	Asthma knowledge & management scales	↑ Asthma knowledge & self-efficacy post intervention	Exemplifies the "delayed intervention" approach; limited by small sample; randomization at school level only
Velsor-Friedrich et al.(2004)	Evaluate an asthma curriculum in 8 inner city schools	Quasi-experimental 2-group design; T=education + 5 home visits, C=UC; pre-, post 2 weeks, 5 months & 12 months	*Open Airways* plus 5 monthly home visits	Small group + single family visits	T=40; C=62; all on public assistance; 69% male; 8–13 y/o	Asthma knowledge, self-efficacy, self-esteem scales, & health indicators	↑ Health outcomes, asthma knowledge & self-esteem by 12-month post intervention	Limited by non-random & small sample; some findings are mixed, but support doing long term support

Notes: T=intervention/treatment group; T1=1st intervention group; T2=2nd intervention group; T3=3rd intervention group; C=control or comparison group; UC=usual care (e.g., physician visit, medication); MFG=multi-family group; ED=Emergency Department.

Implications for Practice and Future Research

On the one hand, according to the findings of systematic review, a comparatively small number of evidence-based interventions in pediatric asthma are available in the literature. Notably, however, given the prevalence of pediatric asthma among minority and poor populations, most of the interventions noted in this chapter were implemented with minority, urban, and/or poorer asthmatic children, and youth, and samples from racial and ethnic populations having asthma. Further, the studies occurred in many settings, any of which is appropriate for social work practice. In sum, these factors substantiate the appropriateness of the interventions for social work practice herein discussed, and the opportunity for social workers to meet more effectively the needs of families with asthmatic children, particularly given the profession's commitment to vulnerable and at-risk populations.

Lastly, one intervention providing promising effectiveness with other chronic illnesses is worth noting here: motivational interviewing. While evaluative research on the effectiveness of motivational interviewing (MI) with some other health disorders are available in the literature (e.g., Channon, Smith, & Gregory, 2003; Smith-West, DiLillo, Bursac, Gore, & Greene, 2007; Stotts, Schmitz, Rhoades, & Grabowski, 2001), only one study of motivational interviewing and asthma was located in this systematic review (Schmaling, Blume, & Afari, 2001). While Borrelli, Riekert, Weinstein, and Rathier (2007) posit the utility of MI as applicable to asthma, unfortunately, the Schmaling et al. study was on asthmatic adults, and, thus, not included in the present chapter. Nonetheless, the demonstrated effectiveness of motivational interviewing in other health disorders certainly suggests that social work practitioners develop, utilize, and evaluate this strategy with asthmatic children.

In summary, the findings of the systematic review on evidence for interventions in this area suggest three opportunities for social workers. One opportunity is to replicate the interventions found to be efficacious. A second opportunity is to replicate the evaluative designs of these studies while also providing interventions with existing promise of effectiveness. The third opportunity is to evaluate the efficacy of motivational interviewing with asthmatic children, teens, and their families to build upon the evidence of this intervention. Thus, the profession can meet the ethical standard of the profession to provide the best practices available to clients, and to advance our knowledge of the best practices for families and their asthmatic children and adolescents.

Glossary

Asthma—a chronic disease of the bronchial tubes (i.e., the airways of the lungs) characterized by tightening of these airways.

Asthma trigger—a dust, animal, pollen, or other element that prompts an asthmatic attack.

Bronchial tubes/bronchi—the tubes, or airways, leading from throat into the lungs.

Bronchospasm—a constriction or tightness of the bronchial tubes.

Chronic illness—an illness that is a serious, ongoing health condition, has a biological, anatomical, or physiologic basis and has lasted, or is expected to last, at least one year.

Co-morbid/co-morbidities—conditions or diseases that are associated with another disease or condition.

Epidemiology—the study of the frequency and distribution of diseases and disease patterns taking into account variations in geography, demographics, socioeconomic status, and genetics.

Etiology—the cause or causes of a disease or abnormal condition as well as the branch of medical science dealing with the causes and origin of diseases.

Incidence—the number of newly diagnosed cases of a disease within a period of time (e.g., year/month, etc.).

Inhalant—a medication in a vaporized form that is taken by breathing the vapor into the bronchi; sometimes these are emergency medications for asthma exacerbations and some are routine medications.

Medically under-served—persons who do not receive adequate or needed medical care due to an absence of available medical care, or to barriers to preventing them accessing health care services.

Morbidity—any departure, subjective or objective, from a state of physical or psychological well being, may be expressed as a proportion of persons per 100,000 persons with a particular diagnosis or condition.

Mortality—the number of deaths in a given year per 100,000 persons in a defined population; the measure of the occurrence of death in a defined population during a specified interval of time.

Prevalence—the proportion of a population having a disease, diagnosis, or medical condition over a specific period (e.g., year) expressed in a percentage.

Risk factor—an established direct cause of, or contributor to, the morbidity or mortality of a particular diagnosis or medical condition.

Sequela(ae)—an after effect of a disease, injury, procedure, or treatment.

Under-insured—having only major medical insurance, or having less than full coverage.

Uninsured—having no health care insurance coverage.

A Scenario for Asthma in Childhood and Adolescence and Questions for Reflection and Discussion

Eleven-year-old José has asthma; he was diagnosed when nine years old. José and his family legally emigrated from Mexico to a major urban area in the U.S., where they currently reside, nearly three years ago. He, and his younger sister and older brother, are fluent in both their native language and English while his mother speaks only Spanish, and his father speaks a little English. José is currently in the fourth grade; his academic performance is generally within the expected range for his grade. During the past two months, however, José has been absent from school at least every two weeks due to exacerbations in his asthma with multiple visits to the emergency room and one hospitalization. José's father has consistent, though low-paid employment that lacks benefits and that frequently requires him to be out of town overnight. José's teacher describes him as a generally happy child, who is enthusiastic about school and seems to have good relationships with the other bilingual children in his class. She does have concerns about his absences; she reports that she hasn't met either of his parents, but has had several conversations with his older brother (sixth grader in the same school as José), who recently told her he thought that his mother was going to have a baby. When asked if there was a plan for the school's participation in insuring vigilance of environmental stressors, information about asthma and José's medication, the teacher responded that she did not think so. José has no medical conditions other than asthma; he takes an oral medication from the school nurse when he arrives at school every morning. The teacher reports that the school nurse said that José was on some form of medical coverages assistance, as the family has no health insurance coverage.

1) What are the challenges for José in completing his current developmental tasks?
2) a) What are the psychosocial stressors influencing José and his family at the present time?
    b) What strategies might be helpful in assisting their coping and adjustment to these stressors?
    c) What information/knowledge would you share with José's family concerning genetics and environmental triggers?
3) How would you collaborate with José's teacher and school personnel and his family to enhance control of his asthma?
4) a) How would your responses to each of the above vary were José to be a female, African American with asthma?
    b) How would you respond differently, or not, were José instead of being 11 years of age, were 14 years of age?

5) What intervention or interventions would you select for work with José and/or his family in the original scenario and in its revisions (i.e., #4 above)?

6) a) What intervention or interventions would you implement with the school on behalf of José?

   b) What intervention or interventions would you implement with the school on behalf of the other students with pediatric asthma?

2   Diabetes

- ◆ Who is affected by diabetes?
- ◆ What is diabetes? What are diabetes medical regimens, and treatments?
- ◆ What are the psycho-social stressors associated with diabetes?
- ◆ What interventions are promising for social work implementation?
  - • For families, adolescents, and children
  - • For adults
- ◆ Glossary
- ◆ Scenario

Introduction

Having diabetes creates a lifelong trajectory of negative effects physically, and psychosocially. In some sense, because of the severity of the possible associated physical conditions and the demands of management, diabetes is the quintessential chronic illness. Practitioners in a variety of settings are likely to encounter clients with diabetes from across the lifespan. This chapter provides the available best practices for psychosocial interventions found to promise efficacy in this work. As with other illnesses discussed in this text, effective practice requires knowledge of the prevalence, and the disease itself, in addition to the psychosocial stressors attendant to the disease. Thus, this chapter discusses the prevalence of diabetes, and the condition and the behavioral and psychosocial factors of having diabetes. Following this discussion, the 20 studies evaluating interventions identified in the present systematic review study and that met the criteria of the present research are explicated. Last, implications for practice and future research, a glossary of relevant terms, and a scenario for discussion conclude the chapter.

Who is Affected by Diabetes?

Diabetes is the fifth leading cause of death in the U.S. (American Diabetes Association, 2005; National Diabetes Information Clearinghouse, 2005). Overall, it is estimated that nearly 24 million (7.8 percent) Americans have diabetes. Of that staggering number, nearly 18 million have already been diagnosed, and the remainder is yet to be diagnosed (American Diabetes Association, 2005). The American Diabetes Association (ADA) reports that the financial cost of diabetes in the U.S. is 132 billion dollars—or one of about every ten dollars spent on health care in America—annually (2005).

Disparities among ethnic and racial groups as indicated by the prevalence rates among ethnic and racial populations is evident. For example, American Natives with a prevalence rate of nearly 15 percent of the Native population are three times more likely to have diabetes than non-Hispanic whites. In fact, one tribe in the west 50 percent of adults between 30 and 64 years of age has diabetes (ADA, 2005; National Diabetes Information Clearinghouse, 2005). African Americans are nearly twice as likely to have diabetes, as are non-Hispanic whites. One-quarter of all older African Americans (65–74 y/o) have diabetes (ADA, 2005; National Diabetes Information Clearinghouse, 2005). The following prevalence rates of diabetes for adult ethnic and racial groups in the U.S. are notable (ADA, 2005):

- Latino Americans: over one and one-half times more likely to have diabetes,
- Mexican Americans: nearly one-quarter have diabetes diagnosis,
- African Americans: diabetes prevalence rate of 11.4 percent.

Diabetes prevalence rates also vary by gender within racial groups. That is, the rate of Type 2 diabetes for adult African American women is nearly twice, and the mortality rate 40 percent higher, than for non-Hispanic white women (Auslander, Haire-Joshu, Houston, Rhee, & Williams, 2002). One-quarter of all African American women have diabetes (ADA, 2005). Vincent and co-authors note that persons of the Latino population have disproportionate prevalence rates of diabetes (Vincent, Pasvogel, & Barrera, 2007). That is, the overall prevalence rate for this population is 10 percent; the prevalence among Latinos 50 years of age and older is reported at 25 to 30 percent. Additionally, these disparities may also reflect culturally related health beliefs, nutritional preferences, and/or genetic factors (Bertera, 2003; Cornelius, 2000; Stern, Gonzalez, Mitchell, Villalpando, Haffner, & Hazuda, 1992; Sudha & Multran, 2001.) Not surprising to professionals, these disparate rates in ethnic and racial groups reflect the disparities in health status related to being poorer, a minority, living with inadequate housing, and other environmental inadequacies.

What is Diabetes?

Diabetes is a disorder of metabolism. That is, diabetes is a disorder of the body's ability to utilize use glucose (sugar) in the bloodstream; glucose is the main source of fuel for the body's functions. After food is digested, the sugar from that food passes into the bloodstream. In the process, the pancreas produces insulin; insulin moves glucose into the cells; glucose is the fuel providing energy and repair at the cellular level.

The production of insulin in the pancreas of persons with diabetes is produced either insufficiently or the insulin produced is sufficient but is ineffective in moving glucose into cells. In these instances, glucose builds up in the blood and does not enter the cells, which are then starved for the nutrition. Thus, then other systems of the body must provide energy for the body's functions.

There are two types of diabetes:

- Type 1
- Type 2

Type 1 diabetes is one of many autoimmune disorders. These disorders result when instead of fighting infections, the body's response turns against itself. In this instance, the body turns its defense mechanisms against the cells in the pancreas that produce insulin (beta cells). Insulin is the hormone that regulates the movement from the bloodstream into cells. Resultantly, where there is insufficient insulin, the normal regulation of the transmission of glucose into cells does not occur. Persons with Type 1 must take insulin, either orally or by injection, to make up for the deficit in their own production of insulin. Another term for Type 1 is "insulin-dependent diabetes." Type 1 diabetes is less prevalent than Type 2, comprising less than 10 percent of all diagnosed diabetics (ADA, 2005).

Type 1 symptoms include increased urination and thirst, continual hunger, weight loss, blurred vision, and fatigue; the symptoms can develop quite rapidly. Type 1 generally develops in children and teens, though it can develop later in life. When not diagnosed or treated, Type 1 diagnosis can develop into a life-threatening coma (i.e., diabetic ketoacidosis). Most researchers believe that the cause of Type 1 is a combination of factors (e.g., Espinet, Osmick, Ahmend, & Villagra, 2005) as follows:

- inactivity,
- obesity,
- propensity to autoimmune disease,
- genetics,
- environmental factors,
- and possibly viruses.

Type 2 diabetes, the most common type of the disorder (an estimated 80–90 percent of diabetes), is also an autoimmune disorder of metabolism.

Type 2 is associated with particular risk factors, including obesity, older age, a family history of diabetes, previous gestational diabetes, a lack of physical activity, and ethnicity (ADA, 2005; National Diabetes Information Clearinghouse, 2005). In contrast to Type 1, Type 2 diabetes, sometimes referred to as non-insulin-dependent diabetes, results from cells being resistant to the actions of insulin, thus glucose does not move from the blood into the cells.

Uncontrolled diabetes of either type has several long-term, relatively minor, and/or potentially life-threatening sequelae. These sequelae are:

- weight loss,
- retinal damage leading to blindness,
- severe skin ulcerations,
- amputations resulting from impaired circulation, kidney damage, coma, and death,
- hardening of the arteries,
- heart disease,
- hypertension.

Some of these sequelae are also disproportionately distributed among racial and/or ethnic groups. For instance, diabetics across all minority groups are at greater risk for early stage kidney disease resulting from diabetes than are non-Hispanic white diabetics (Centers for Disease Control & Prevention, 2006a). Some of the complication rates among racially diverse populations compared to non-Hispanic white diabetics differ dramatically (ADA, 2005). For example,

- Mexican American diabetics are 4.5 to 6.6 times as likely to have end stage renal disease,
- amputation of lower limbs for First Nations Peoples with diabetes is 3–4 times more likely,
- African American diabetics are twice as likely to have diabetes-related retinopathy.

It is likely that social and economic disparities underlie these variations by cultural background, race, and ethnicity, such as access to health care, insurance status, the health-related effects of poverty (Sudha & Multran, 2001). Some authors also suggest a linkage between diabetes and culturally-linked health beliefs about the disease, nutrition, and/or mainstream versus alternative health care (Bertera, 2003; Cornelius, 2000; Kaiser Family Foundation, 2004; Lorig, Ritter, & Jacquez, 2005; Philis-Tsimikas & Walker, 2001).

Societal and personal costs due to the increased cost of diabetes-related disability, morbidity, and mortality are burdensome for individuals, families, and society. The financial cost of diabetes for individuals and families is extensive due to the need for ongoing and consistent medical care to avoid the negative sequelae of the disease. The financial cost of diabetes in the U.S. in 2002 was 132 billion dollars (direct and indirect costs combining disability, work loss, premature mortality, etc.) (ADA, 2005).

Diabetes also poses a heavy psychosocial and lifestyle encumbrance on persons with diabetes and on their families. Not only are persons with diabetes Type 2 likely to have the physical sequelae of the disorder, as noted above, they also experience disruptions in daily lives, and required alterations in lifestyle. These emotional, behavioral, and psychosocial problems in relation to children and adolescents, and their families, and subsequently to adults with diabetes are discussed below.

Psychosocial Impact and Stressors of Diabetes

Children and Adolescents

The emotional and social impact on children and teens, and their families, is related to the age of onset and to the extent of necessary treatment for the child. In general, treatment for either type of diabetes incorporates a nutritional regime, often medications (pill or injectable), management of physical activity, daily decision-making, and behavioral changes to control the disease effectively. For children and teens, the challenges of psychosocial and physical developmental tasks and adjustments, adhering to diet and to medications is difficult. The responsibilities of families, particularly for families with children or teens having Type 1 diabetes, are continual and only somewhat lessened for families with offspring with Type 2 diabetes (Anderson, Loughlin, Goldberg, & Laffel, 2001; Bertera, 2003).

Anderson and co-authors (2001) note that families being overwhelmed and burning out on the tasks of diabetes management is of concern in the professional literature. In their long-term study of the concerns of families about their diabetic children, three specific major concerns emerged. These were:

- how the disease may affect their child's behavior at the current time,
- how the disease may change the family and parent's interactions with the child,
- how the disease can produce tension in the family.

These concerns are very understandable given the magnitude of the medical regimens required to control Type 1 diabetes effectively. According to Anderson and colleagues (2001), these concerns converge with the longer-term worry of how the disease will affect their child's psychosocial and physical health, and well-being in the future. The convergent worries understandably prompt family members' anxiety, fear, and guilt over how well they will be able to manage their child's diabetes, and ensure their future well-being.

Coupled with those anxieties are the family's daily responsibilities for diabetes management. These include specific monitoring of blood glucose levels, and medications, and nutritional intake and physical activity; each of the latter can affect blood glucose levels, and, thus reciprocally, medication needs (Hoff, Mullins, Gillaspy, Page, Pelt, & Chaney, 2005). Families balance the task to controlling glucose levels to prevent both hypoglycemic blood levels with its negative outcomes (unconsciousness and seizures), and extremely high glucose levels (hyperglycemic) with its negative outcomes (nerve damage, blindness, kidney damage), and their child's normative daily lifestyle and developmental needs.

In sum, managing a child's diabetes influences the family's life, siblings, parent–child interactions and the well-being of the family over-all. Parents must appropriately address any unexpected complications of their child's diabetes-related and resultant need for health care services. The characteristics of Type 1 diabetes may pose risk factors for parents and caretakers intensifying their psychosocial stress related to having a child with diabetes. These are reported to include anxiety, depressive symptoms, sleep problems and/or somatization (Hoff et al., 2005).

Some research findings suggest that family structure, and race or ethnicity may be related to ineffective management of pediatric diabetes. Thompson, Auslander, and White (2001) examined family structural and the health of adolescents with Type 1 diabetes in a convenience sample of 155 diabetic teens and their mothers. Findings from in-person interviews and questionnaires (e.g., demographics and family character-istics), and blood glucose level monitoring suggest that teen diabetics of single-parent families were in poorer health and, specifically, had more poorly controlled blood glucose levels. Thompson and co-authors note that single-parent families also were more likely to be of minority status and of lower SEC. The implications of these factors and effectively managing children's diabetes, and the psychosocial stressors associated with the disorder are typical of associations with other chronic illnesses, as well.

Cultural background and related health beliefs concerning eating habits, nutrition, and spiritually-based beliefs about individual responsi-bility for health are reported to challenge both the dietary requirements for treating diabetes, and adherence to the medication regimens, both of which are necessary for effective control of diabetes (Auslander, et al., 2002; DeCoster, 2003; DeCoster & Cummings, 2004). For example, it is suggested that the significantly higher rate of diabetes in African Americans may be linked to the greater amount of fat in their traditional diet compared to non-Hispanic whites, even after controlling for other risk factors (Auslander et al., 2002).

Stressors for adults with diabetes arise largely from the nature of the disorder being a chronic illness, including the lifelong need to adapt behaviorally to the illness itself, and to the daily regimens required to control the disease (McQuaid & Nassau, 1999). These daily stressors can be exacerbated by recurrent interruptions in routine health care, and may be lessened by effective social support systems (Karlsen, Idsoe, Hanestad, Murberg, & Bru, 2004). Karlsen et al. explored the relationships among these elements of living with diabetes in a sample of 587 adult diabetics (2004). Several outcome measures were used to assess support and perceptions of support from family members, health care providers and peers, as well as standardized diabetes-related stress, coping styles, depression, and anxiety scales. Of particular relevance to the social work ecological perspective is their finding concerning the centrality of the family of the adult diabetic in both exacerbating stress when family relationships are negative or conflicted, and facilitating coping by the diabetic when family interactions are positive. The current systematic review located a total of 20 studies that met the criteria for inclusion. These are discussed below.

Promising Interventions with Children and Adolescent Diabetics, and Parents

Children and teens with diabetes most often have Type 1. Possibly because this type of diabetes can be more difficult to control, and due to the potential severity of physical, psychosocial, and emotional consequences on the diabetic, and on their families, the research in this area has accumulated several promising interventions. The studies located in the present research evaluated interventions with families, children, adolescents, and adult diabetics.

Promising Family-Centered Interventions

Three evaluations among those located in this systematic review were family-centered interventions. In fact, the majority of evaluations focused on adolescents and children with diabetes were family-centered interventions. This finding reflects the increasing knowledge that the family system is central in managing the diabetes of youth and children.

Wysocki et al. (2000) evaluated the effect of behavioral family systems therapy (BFST) with families experiencing conflict over their teen's diabetes, and their Type 1 diabetic adolescents in an RCT study three group design, with baseline, post-intervention and two follow-up outcome measures (i.e., post three, six and 12 months). Participants (n = 118) were randomly assigned to usual health care (C = 32), or to ten sessions of BFST (T1 = 36), or to ten sessions of a multi-family educational support group (T2 = 36). The majority of participating families were white; teen diabetics were between 12 and 17 years of age, on average being 16.8 years old. Behavioral family systems therapy is a combination of cognitive behavioral therapy (e.g., contracting, modeling, communication patterns, and modeling) and family systems therapy (e.g., intervening on weak parental coalitions, cross-generational coalitions). Measurements included three validated scales measuring family structure, conflict and diabetes related conflict, Self-Care Inventory completed by the teen diabetic and glucose levels. The researchers report families in the BFST group evidenced improved family relationships and reduced conflict at each post-intervention point. No differences were found in diabetic control of the adolescents. Nonetheless, these findings lend support to the use of behavioral family therapy with adolescents with Type 1 diabetes. The authors report extensive details of the interventions as well as the design, and data analysis, thus, providing practitioners with necessary information for replication of the intervention and of the evaluation plan.

More recently, Wysocki and fellow researchers (2007) continued their RCT evaluation of BFST with adolescents with Type 1 diabetes and their families. The study specifically sought to evaluate further the intervention's effect on glycemic control of the adolescents. Outcome measures, therefore, included family conflict, patterns, and dynamics as in their earlier work, as well as treatment adherence and glycemic control; measurement points occurring at baseline, post-six, 12, and 18 months. The sample of 104 families of adolescent diabetics were randomly assigned to usual care (C = 32), or to 12 sessions of a multi-family educational support group (T1 = 36), or to 12 sessions of BFST (T2 = 36). Analysis of data showed that a significantly higher proportion of youth in the BFST group adhered to their diabetic regiment and control of their blood glucose levels at each measurement point. The findings on measurements on family conflicts were mixed, with some improvement shown in both treatment interventions.

A random controlled trial evaluated an intervention with parents of newly diagnosed children (under 18 years of age) implemented and evaluated by Hoff et al. (2005). The intervention targeted parental uncertainty and distress, and their child's behavioral problems, centering on teaching parents skills to manage uncertainty. Participating families were randomly assigned to the intervention (n = 25) or usual care (n = 21) groups in the pre-test, post one-month, and post-six month design. Outcome measures were on diabetes related distress, uncertainty, and child behavior problems (i.e., CBCL). Significant reductions in the parent distress measures and ratings of their child's behavior problems were found in the intervention group compared with the control group. The centrality of the family in monitoring their child's Type 1 diabetes and their ability to effectively cope with the unknowns of the diagnosis and its trajectory support the inclusion here of this study despite the small sample size. Further, the authors provide extensive details of the intervention.

Overall, these interventions for family-centered interventions with diabetic children and youth provide some promise for intervening at the family level. This promise is limited, however, given the small sample sizes of the three studies.

Interventions with Adolescents

Four promising interventions with diabetic adolescents that met all the criteria of the review were located. The following discussion begins with two RCT studies using small group interventions, and is followed by discussion of the two studies evaluating motivational interviewing in individual sessions with diabetic teens.

Recently Ellis and colleagues evaluated the efficacy of a six-month multi-systemic therapy (MST) intervention with adolescents with poorly controlled diabetes (Type 1) who received their medical care for diabetes at a university hospital (Ellis, Frey, Naar-King, Templin, Cunningham, & Cakan, 2005). The RCT study evaluated the effect of MST on stress related to the teens' diabetes in a baseline and post-intervention and post-six month follow up design. Participants were randomly assigned to the intervention group or to usual care. Their findings demonstrated that the intervention significantly reduced family stress, and increased diabetes control.

Grey and co-researchers evaluated an intervention on coping skills training to improve control of diabetes and enhance quality of life in adolescents with Type 1 diabetes in a university's diabetic clinic for children and youth (Grey, Boland, Davidson, Ma, Sullivan-Bolyai, & Tamborlane, 1998). The RCT two-group comparison group design with baseline and post-intervention measures randomly assigned teens to an intervention that combined intensive management plus coping skills training (CST) or the intensive management without CST (control). The adolescents were 13 to 20 years of age, all female, and nearly all non-Hispanic white, 34 of whom were in the intervention group and 31 in the control group. CST is a series of small group sessions focusing on coping skills, cognitive behavior medication, and conflict resolution. Outcome measures included general self-efficacy, diabetes self-efficacy, coping depression, quality of life scales, glucose monitoring, and use of injected insulin (as indicators of glucose control). The combined CST intervention was effective in controlling blood glucose levels to optimum target balanced levels, and increasing the self-efficacy, and coping. However, no significant post-intervention (three months) change was found in diabetes life satisfaction, diabetic worries, or the depression scales. Of note are the details provided of the CST intervention facilitating replication by practitioners.

A very early pre-post- and follow-up designed study evaluated an intervention with children and their parents in separate small group sessions with voluntary participants in an intervention group and a control group. A total of 14 (nine to 13 years of age) insulin-dependent children and at least one of each of their parents participated (Gross, Magalinck, & Richardson, 1985). The intervention for the children's group and for the parent's group focused on self-management training, incorporating information on Type 1 diabetes, and behavior modification of children's behavior to reduce family conflict and to improve the children's maintenance of glucose levels. Multiple baselines pre- and post-tests included scales for parental assessment of children's behavioral changes in diabetic self-management, and family conflict. Daily logs completed by the parents were required noting self-management behaviors of the children. Findings imply that, though limited by the small sample size and the absence of validated instruments, the intervention reduced the frequency and severity of family conflicts related to the child's diabetes at post-test points and at follow-up six months later.

Motivational Interviewing in Interventions with Adolescent Diabetics

The efficacy of motivational interviewing (MI) is receiving support in regard to various health issues, including drug abuse, alcoholism, and psychiatric dual diagnosis (e.g., Baker, Boggs, & Lewin, 2001; Knight, McGowan, Dickens, & Bundy, 2006; Rubak, Sandboek, Lauritzen, & Christensen, 2005; Stotts et al., 2001). MI is a short-term intervention strategy designed as a practitioner directive, client-centered approach to promoting behavior change based on problem solving and cognitive behavior change approaches, and that supports of self-efficacy (Emmons & Rollnick, 2001). Specific techniques in using MI are motivating the client, clearly developing an agenda for the work, resolving ambivalence, goal setting, rephrasing and reframing, and reflection to name just a few (Borrelli et al., 2007). Golay, Lagger, Chambouleyron, Carrard, and Lasserre-Moutet (2008) delineate the purposes, the therapeutic relationship, and specific techniques of motivational interviewing and apply these to health care education with patients. The overall purpose of MI is described as a way to assist clients in helping themselves, through sharing decisions concerning health, and achieving goals for better health with the client/patient. Golay and co-authors discussions of specific techniques including negotiating, role playing, actions, and working through relapses in a clear and cogent manner. Lastly, the authors apply and explicate MI with a fictional client with Type 2 diabetes.

Clearly, this approach is appropriate for social workers for intervening in the psychosocial and behavioral components of effectively living with diabetes. Recently, interest increased in evaluating MI for outcome changes in specific health disorders, including diabetes. Two such studies of motivational interviewing with adolescents with Type 1 diabetes were located in the present research. These studies are by Viner and colleagues (2003), and a second is by Channon and colleagues (2007).

Viner, Christie, Taylor, and Hey (2003) implemented a combined small group intervention with adolescents aged 11 to 17 years of age with poorly controlled diabetes Type 1. Teen volunteers, whose parents gave consent, were divided into two age groups: 10 to 13 and 14 to 17 years of age, and matched by gender, SEC, and duration of their diabetes. These adolescents were assigned to either the treatment group (n-21), while teens who opted out of the intervention, most often due to non-availability for the weekly sessions, became the control group (n = 56). The six-weekly session intervention was evaluated at post-intervention, one to three months, four to six, and seven to 12 months post-intervention with outcome measures on diabetic management indicators (e.g., insulin use, glucose levels, etc.), and a diabetes related stress index.

The small group intervention combined motivational interviewing and solution focused brief therapy. As discussed clearly by the researchers, MI focuses on moving the client through the several stages (i.e., pre-contemplation, contemplation, preparation, action, and maintenance); later stages are seen as more motivating in achieving the client's goals. Solution-focused therapy seeks to work with the client to identify those behaviors that are beneficial, and those that are not beneficial in reaching goals. Targets in terms Viner et al.'s study were control of blood glucose, diabetic symptomology and diabetes related stress. Blood glucose levels over the post-intervention measurement points were significantly improved in the intervention group compared with the control group, and were maintained at later measurement points for a majority of the treatment group participants who also had reduced levels of diabetes-related distress at the post-intervention measurement points. The efficacy of the intervention, however, is limited due to the non-randomization, voluntary participation, and the small size of the sample.

Channon and co-authors report an evaluation of an RCT effective-ness study on motivational interviewing with 66 adolescents with Type 1 diabetes, who were randomly assigned to the intervention group or the control group (usual care) with baseline, six, 12, and 24 month outcome measurement points (Channon, Huws-Thomas, Rollnick, Cannings-John, Rogers, & Gregory, 2007). Participants in the interven-tion group received individual sessions with motivation interviewing (MI) over a one-year period. The researchers utilized the same measurement tools as those of Grey et al. (1998) and report significant differences between the intervention and the control groups at 12 months, including higher diabetes life satisfaction, and lower worries and anxiety scores in the intervention group. In a post-24 month follow-up these improve-ments were maintained, suggesting that long-term change through MI interventions has promise of efficacy.

Promising Interventions with Children

As presented above, recent studies involving children with diabetes are primarily family-centered interventions, rather than individual interventions directly with children. Only one evaluation of intervening directly with children that met the current criteria was located in this systematic review.

An intervention to evaluate the effect of an educational program with children with Type 1 diabetes targeted diabetic self-care skills and knowledge among eight- to 12-year-old diabetic children in a pediatric clinic of a children's hospital (McNabb, Quinn, Murphy, Thorp, & Cook, 1995). The age group was selected as developmentally appropriate for children to begin to share responsibility with their parents over the management of their diabetes. Potential participant children were volunteered by their parents; these children were screened for appropriateness, and informed parental consent elicited. Twenty-two children met eligibility requirements and had parental consent (T = 10; C = 12). Those in the control group received their usual medical care at the clinic.

The intervention group of children participated in six, small group, one-hour, weekly sessions focused on knowledge of diabetes, and independence in self-care skills (e.g., symptom identification and communication, glucose levels, insulin use). Parents completed scales on a weekly basis measuring each element of the management skills on the extent that they had observed their child's independence. Evaluation at post-test of the children's independent responsibility for self-care revealed significant improvements on each outcome measure. These findings are limited, of course, by the small sample size, the method of recruitment, and the possibility that parents may have exaggerated their child's independence. However, this very early study is supportive of intervening directly with young children in facilitating their effective management of diabetes Type 1. (See Table 2.1 for summarizations of the studies discussed above.)

In brief, though diabetes in children and youth is largely Type 1, a plethora of efficacious interventions with this population is not available in the literature. On the one hand, this finding is disheartening. On the other hand, two of the interventions for direct practice with adolescent diabetics themselves using motivational interviewing was located. This finding is hopeful as the intervention is widely evaluated in relation to other health disorders, and found to be efficacious for many. Practitioners working with diabetic adolescents in particular are encouraged to implement the techniques and approach of motivational interviewing with their clients.

Promising Interventions with Adult Diabetics

Over a majority of diabetics are adults with Type 2 diabetes, the most common type of diabetes. Thus, it is not surprising that the majority of

Table 2.1 Interventions with families, and diabetic children and adolescents

Author (year)	Objective	Design	Intervention	Mode	Sample	Outcome measures	Results	Notes
Channon et al. (2007)	Evaluate the efficacy of MI with teens with Type 1 in diabetic clinics	RCT 2-group, baseline, post-12 & 24 months design	T = MI over 12 months; C = support only	Individual	T = 38, C = 24; all white, middle SEC	Glucose monitoring, DM QOL, Knowledge, & Self-efficacy, Child Locus of Health Control, Well-being, & Family Behavior scales	T = ↓ glucose levels & ↑ psychosocial measures at each post-test point compared to C group	Provides details of MI use & design; applies MI to younger sample with positive results
Ellis et al. (2005)	Evaluate MST with poor controlled DM teens	RCT, 2-group, pre-post design; T = MST; C = UC	MST weekly over 6 months on family stress levels, & control of DM; MST addresses family, ecological processes	Individual	N = 127; no other details provided	Stress, DM control, treatment adherence, & hospitalizations	T ↓ stress, use of hospitals & ↑ control of DM & DM adherence	MST is seen as effective with teens with other problems; absence of details is limiting
Grey et al. (1998)	Evaluate coping skills training (CST) in teens with poorly controlled DM Type 1	RCT, 2-group, pre-post design; T = CST + UC; C = UC alone	CST is a small group intervention on coping with DM, using CBT, & insulin use	Small group	T = 34; C = 31; all female & white, 13–20 y/os	Self-efficacy & life satisfaction re: DM, coping in DM, & QOL scales; glucose & insulin use monitoring	T = optimal DM control achieved at post & post-test; ↑ DM self-efficacy & satisfaction; no other changes	Small sample; creative approach to teens having difficulty in managing DM

(continued)

Table 2.1 Interventions with families, and diabetic children and adolescents *(continued)*

Author (year)	Objective	Design	Intervention	Mode	Sample	Outcome measures	Results	Notes
Gross et al. (1985)	Evaluate with multiple baseline design intervention on DM related family conflict & DM control	2-group comparison design with a convenience & multiple baseline & post-measurement design	T = manual on DM control, family conflict, behavior modification skills, & DM self-management; 1½ hour weekly sessions for 8 weeks. C = UC	Small group; parent & child separate groups	14 children with DM; aged 9–13 years, & 1 or both parents T = 7 & C = 7	Parent completed family conflicts, child behavior & glucose logs, behavior rating scales	Graphs show that T group had steadily ↓ conflict & ↑ behaviors & glucose control	Very small sample; shows use of multiple baseline studies easily replicated
Hoff et al. (2005)	Evaluate parent intervention with children newly diagnosed DB in 2 diabetes clinics	RCT 2-group, pre/post, post-1 & post 6 month follow-up design; T = intervention; C = UC	2 sessions (2.5 hrs. each) on weekends on parental distress & uncertainty re: DM diagnosis, the dynamics, management, resources on DM Type 1	Small group	T = 25, C = 21 families, all white; child less than 18 y/o; T = 41% & C = 53% girls; all children Type 1	PPUS- uncertainty re: child's illness; SCL-90- distress; BASC/PRS- parent assessment of child's adaptive & problem behaviors	T ↓ PPUS, SCL-90 & PRS compared to C at each post-test	A small pilot study addressing the stress of new DM diagnosis in children
McNabb et al. (1995)	Evaluate education program in pediatric clinic on DM self-care in Type 1 children	RCT pre-post, matched group design; matched by age & race; Control = UC	Six 1 hour sessions on diabetic knowledge & self-care skills shaped to age of children (8–12 years old)	Small group	T = 10; aged 9.7 years; C = 12; aged 10.0 years	Glucose levels, self-care skills & knowledge	T ↑ self-care of DM at post tests; no differences in glycemic control between T & C	Small sample; not often studied age group

Author (Year)	Purpose	Design	Intervention	Format/Setting	Sample	Measures	Findings	Comments
Viner et al. (2003)	Evaluate combined approach with teens with poorly controlled DM in 4 urban DM clinics	Non-random, controlled, 2-group, pre-test & post-test 4, 6 & 12- month design; groups formed by age (10–13 y/o & 14-17 y/os)	T = MI + SFT; C = UC	Small group	14–17 y/os w/ similar DM histories & glucose at baseline; T = 21 (72% female; C = 21 (40% female)	DM Self-efficacy, Strengths & Difficulties scales, glucose monitoring	T = ↓ improved glucose control & improved psychosocial measures at post-test points compared to C group	Lacking random & small sample; supports use of MI with diabetic teens with poor control of DM, MI + SFT is very detailed
Wysocki et al. (2000)	Evaluate a behavioral family therapy (BFST) with families in conflict re: teen's DM	RCT 3 groups, pre-post + 2 follow-ups; T1 = BFST; T2 = MFG; C = UC	10 sessions of behavioral family therapy BFST or MFG	1:1 family or MFG	C = 32; T1 = 36; T2 = 36; 78% white families; 12–17 y/o teens, average 16.8 years; all Type 1 DM	Parent-Adolescent Conflict, Issue Checklist, DM Conflict scales; DM adherence scale, glucose control	T1 = ↓ family conflict & ↑ cohesiveness over T2 & C; no ↑ glucose control in any group	Small sample, RCT study targeting teens with problems in DM control & family conflict re: DM; extensive details given
Wysocki et al. (2007)	Evaluate BFST-D with families in conflict re: teen's DM	RCT; 3 group, pre-post + 3 follow-ups; T1 = BFST-D +UC; T2 = MFG education +UC; C = UC	12 sessions- BFST-D + UC, or MFG educational sessions + UC; BFST-D is revised BFST	1:1 family, or MFG	T1 61%, T2 = 75%, C = 61% white; all Type 1 DM; ~50% male T1, T2, & C	DM self management scales for adolescents; adherence checklist, and glucose control	T1 = ↑ control of DM & DM adherence over T2 & C at follow up points	Refined 2000 study; details given of design & groups; implies BFST-D in MFG mode worth study

Notes: T = intervention/treatment group; T1 = 1st intervention group; T2 = 2nd intervention group; T3 = 3rd intervention group; C = control or comparison group; UC = usual care (e.g., physician visit, medication); MFG = multi-family group; ED = Emergency Department; DM = diabetes mellitus.

studies located in this systematic review found studies evaluating interventions with these adults. In fact, eleven studies evaluating interventions with adult diabetics were located. The modalities of these interventions included small group, and one-on-one sessions alone or combined with small group sessions.

Gilliland, Azen, Perez, and Carter (2002) conducted a quasi-experimental non-randomized three-group comparison study with diabetic Native American adult diabetics delivered in a community setting. The three-group study assigned participants to two family-centered intervention small groups (T1 and T2) and one control group. Those in the T1 group (n = 32) received ten multi-family group sessions (MFG) plus individual family sessions after the multi-family group sessions concluded. The T2 group (n = 39) received interventions in individual family sessions only with the same content as the MFG modality; and those in the Control group (n = 33) received only usual medical care. The curriculum materials of the intervention (diabetes education, diabetes management skills, and social support) whether delivered in MFG or in one-on-one family sessions were developed previously by the researchers (Carter et al., 1997). The curriculum materials incorporated cultural norms (e.g., foods, lifestyle), folk stories, and values of First Nations Peoples, and social learning theory. Videos in the intervention were developed prior to the research through community focus groups to reflect Native lifestyle, and incorporate Native persons in the video. Findings on pre- and post 12 month data showed that those in the combined intervention (T1) had significantly lower blood sugar levels and greater weight loss over the one-year period. The import of the intervention's promise of efficacy relates to the disproportionate rate of diabetes among this population. Notably, the authors provide detail about the content of the educational and lifestyle interventions, and about the developmental processes used to produce culturally sensitive content, thus, speaking to the bio-psych-social environmental context of social work and to practice with Natives and other cultural groups.

Vincent et al. (2007) conducted a study of a culturally tailored intervention with Mexican American adults with Type 2 diabetes in a pretest/posttest RCT two-group study (T1 = 10; C = 7) with a convenience sample (71 percent female aged 37–69 years of age). The intervention (T1) occurred in a community center on the reservation and focused on disease management skills for chronic illness to increased self-efficacy and diabetic self-management skills (e.g., medication adherence, physical activity, glucose monitoring). Vincent and colleagues report that the intervention resulted in positive clinical and statistical outcomes in diabetes knowledge, weight control, body mass index measures, and improvements in self-efficacy at post-intervention points. Though the findings are limited by the very small sample size, the study, and its findings have relevance for social work in its shaping the intervention for Mexican American adults, and improved outcomes for a population whose prevalence rate of diabetes is very high (i.e., 25 percent).

An RCT study of a patient education intervention with adult participants with Type 2 diabetes by Adolfsson, Walker-Engstrom, Smide, and Wikblad (2007) included a one-year follow-up conducted in seven primary care centers in Sweden. The authors report that the empowerment small group educational intervention focused on diabetes knowledge and self-efficacy, and glucose control. The participants were randomly assigned to the control group (n = 46) and received only usual medical care or to the treatment group (n = 46). Pre-intervention and post-intervention at one-year follow-up measures were completed covering diabetic knowledge and self-efficacy, satisfaction with daily life and medical indicators of diabetes (e.g., glycemic control). At one-year follow-up, the intervention group had significantly greater diabetes knowledge and maintained better glycemic control than the control group. However, no differences were found in satisfaction or self-efficacy. Useful details of the small group intervention are provided facilitating replication of the intervention and the study.

Attention in developing efficacious interventions for specific ethnic and racial populations of adult diabetics is increasing. An example of a random control study with this objective in mind is a group educational plus individual counseling intervention by Gallegos, Ovalle-Berumen, and Gomez-Meza (2006). Though the study involved nursing personnel, the intervention and its psychosocial perspective are clearly appropriate to social work practice. The comparison design with repeated measures (baseline, and every three months for one year) involved one group receiving the combined intervention (n = 25), and the comparison group (n = 20) receiving only usual care.

The combined intervention focused on knowledge of the relationship of having diabetes and overall health, and specific dietary and nutritional management tailored to ethnic preferences and beliefs, as well as blood glucose monitoring, implemented in six sessions of one and one-half hours each over 50 weeks. Psychosocial outcome measurements were Likert scale questionnaires: two diabetic self-management scales, and one scale measuring adaptation to health previously validated among Mexican American diabetic samples, and monitoring of blood glucose levels. Findings included improved blood glucose control, and improved self-care knowledge and adaptation to diabetes at four post-interventions points. Beneficial to the purposes of this text is that the authors detail the intervention and the longer term outcome measurements.

Auslander and colleagues examined the efficacy of a culturally-specific peer led small group educational three-month intervention with African American women being at risk for Type 2 diabetes targeting adaptation to the diabetic nutritional regimen, dietary control (Auslander et al., 2002). The community-based six-session small group randomly assigned intervention was shaped to the stage of change concepts (n = 294; intervention = 138; control = 156), and combined the small group sessions with six individual sessions with participants. Peer educators came from the participants' community and were trained by social workers, and nutritional and health educators. The manual-based intervention centered on diet management skills, knowledge on understanding food and nutritional labels, modifying recipes, as applied to the home and to eating out. Outcome measures taken at baseline, post-test, and follow up were on diabetes related knowledge, attitudes about diet and health, and dietary planning. Of these dietary changes, caloric intake, and food label-reading knowledge were significantly improved in the intervention group. The study demonstrates the utility of community-based peer led interventions, and the import of social work's role in implementing such interventions.

Bradshaw et al. (2007) examined the efficacy of a training approach to increase the psychosocial and physical functioning of adults with Type 2 diabetes through resiliency training. The RCT, baseline, post-three and post-six month designed study assigned patients who had previously participated in a standard self-education program on diabetes (e.g., symptoms, etiology, triggers) to the resiliency intervention (T = 30) or the control (C = 37; usual care) groups. The resiliency intervention was a ten module (15 hour) small group intervention based on a resiliency model aimed at developing self-directed behavior changes. Outcome variables were blood sugar levels, daily diaries of eating and exercise, and scales measuring the psychosocial constructs of self-efficacy, locus of control, social support, and purpose in life. Bradshaw and co-authors report findings supporting the efficacy of the resiliency intervention on the psychosocial outcome measures at both three and six months post intervention. Unexpectedly, no differences were obtained for the intervention on dietary, physical activity, or blood glucose measures. The authors note that, given the centrality of psychosocial variables and their relationship to glycemic control suggested in the literature, the evidence for this intervention is promising.

Empowerment conceptualized as the ability to maintain effective control over, in this case Type 1 diabetes, is pivotal in the long-term management of diabetes and prevention of negative physical and emotional sequelae (Forlani, Zannoni, Tarrini, Melchionda, & Marchesini, 2006). These researchers implemented such an educational intervention to promote active self-care, and well-being in adults with Type 1 diabetes in a non-randomized comparison group study with a convenience sample (T = 55; C = 36). Outcomes were evaluated on the basis of the SF-36, the Psychological General Well Being (PGWB) and a Well Being Enquiry for Diabetics (WED) measurement scales completed at baseline and at 12 months post-intervention. The small group (8–10 members) intervention of eight sessions (two hours each) concentrated on specific diabetes knowledge, dietary requirements, monitoring of blood glucose, coping with diabetes, family, and lifestyle challenges, and strategies for seeking social support. Notably, each of the psychosocial outcomes (i.e., PGWB subscales on anxiety, depression, general well being) and each of the subscales of the SF-36 (e.g., role limitations, vitality, general health, mental health) were significantly improved at post-intervention and at follow up one year later. These findings are constrained, of course, due to the non-random, small sample. However, the authors do provide specific details on the intervention, and the import of the significant changes in psychosocial outcomes.

Anderson, Funnell, Butler, Arnold, Fitzgerald, and Feste (1993) implemented a randomized, waitlist-controlled pre-post evaluation also of an empowerment educational intervention with adult diabetics, who were recruited through advertisements and mailers; volunteers were randomly assigned to the intervention group (n = 23) or to the wait-list control group (n = 22). The empowerment intervention targets goal setting, problem solving, coping with limits of achieving goals, and managing stress in six weekly one-hour sessions. Outcome measurements included blood sugar level reporting, and self-report on five scales measuring diabetes self-efficacy components of the intervention. The empowerment intervention resulted in significantly increased blood glucose control, and increased diabetes self-efficacy scales. These findings are constrained by the small sample size, the absence of standardized measurement scales, and recruitment methods, but do lend some early support for the effect of educational group interventions with diabetic adults.

Motivational Interviewing with Adult Diabetics

As discussed previously in this chapter, the efficacy of motivational interviewing is receiving support concerning several health issues, The following three studies by Greaves and colleagues, and by Smith (1997) and Smith-West and colleagues (2007) implemented MI in their evaluative research.

Greaves and colleagues (2008) in a two-group study with pre-diabetic adults in primary care centers randomly assigned participants to the intervention group or to the comparison group. The intervention group received individual counseling sessions with motivational interviewing techniques (n = 68); the comparison group received only an information booklet (n = 69). Greaves et al. report that achieving the target weight loss (an indicator of risk for diabetes) and increasing physical activity per day was achieved by statistically more participants in the intervention group than in the control group at the six-month post-intervention point.

Smith and co-researchers (1997) evaluated a pilot study with a random assignment, comparison group design. The intervention combined three sessions of individual motivational interviewing within a 16-week weight management program compared to the 16-week weight control program among older diabetic women (41 percent African American; N = 22) (Smith, Heckemeyer, Kratt, & Mason, 1997). Outcome measures were journaling food intake, attendance in the weight management program, and blood glucose levels. Findings demonstrated more consistent food diary journaling, and better maintained blood sugar levels in the intervention group, but no significant differences in weight loss between the two groups. The authors provide details of the intervention and the weight control program, thus facilitating replication of the interventions.

Smith-West and colleagues (2007) replicated the earlier pilot study note above (1997) in an expanded version of the weight management program in a RCT designed study on the efficacy of MI (Smith et al., 1997; Smith-West et al., 2007). Participants (n = 217) were randomly assigned to either the 42 session program plus either five sessions of MI (T = 109) over 12 months or to five attention-placebo sessions of instruction on various topics of health relevant to women (C = 108). Compared to the control group, glycemic control and weight loss were significantly improved in the intervention group at six months, but were not maintained after that point. In brief, both the earlier Smith et al. study (1997) and the recent replication (2007) support the efficacy of MI on weight loss.

The interventions with adult diabetics located in this review are fairly impressive in their use of randomized designs, and motivational interviewing in the specific. These promising interventions should be further developed given the expanding prevalence of diabetes, particularly in minority populations. The details afforded in these studies can prompt practitioners to replicate not only the interventions located as appropriate to their adult clients with diabetes in light of the population's cultural background, goals and values, but also the evaluation designs to substantiate their promise in their own practice. (See Table 2.2 for summaries of the studies discussed above.)

Implications for Practice and Future Research

Clearly, more evidence needs to accrue regarding interventions with diabetic children and their families given the severity of the sequelae and co-morbidities, and the difficulty of effectively controlling Type 1 diabetes. Notwithstanding, these findings of promising practice approaches support practitioners' use of EBP with diabetics. However, one of the challenges for practitioners desiring to implement best practices is the need to match the characteristics of samples in efficacy studies with the characteristics of their own clients and client systems. It is therefore worth noting the need for further research on best practices with more diverse and larger samples of adult, children and adolescent diabetics.

Table 2.2 Interventions with diabetic adults

Author (year)	Objective	Design	Intervention	Mode	Sample	Outcome measures	Results	Notes
Adolfsson et al. (2007)	Evaluate education intervention with adult diabetics in 7 clinics in Sweden	RCT 2-group, pre-post & 1 year follow-up design; T=42; C=UC=46	Empowerment educational intervention on self-management, & self-efficacy in diabetes	Small group	T = 57% male, 2/3 w/ jobs, 83% married average 62 y/o; C=61% male, 2/3 w/job, 2/3 married average 64 y/o	Diabetes knowledge, glycemic control, diabetic self-efficacy	T = ↑diabetes knowledge & glycemic control at post-tests compared to the control group	Small sample with limited findings; useful details of sessions of intervention provided
Anderson et al. (1993)	Evaluate culturally-specific peer intervention with African American diabetic women	RCT 2-group, waitlist control group pre-post, & follow-up	Culturally tailored diabetic nutritional 6 weekly manual-based self-care, diet management led by peers	Small group + 6 single sessions	T = 22 C = 22	Glucose levels, diabetes knowledge, attitudes, beliefs, self-efficacy & diet planning	T ↑ glucose control & diabetes self-efficacy at post test	Small sample. Supports peer educators with African American female diabetics
Auslander et al. (2002)	Evaluate peer led education to reduce risk of diabetes in pre-diabetic African American women	RCT 2-group pre-post & follow up design; T = 138 C = 156	6 sessions on dietary change & skills for control diet	Small group + 6 single person sessions	T = average age 41; 23% married; 47% below poverty line; C=average age 40; 48% below poverty line	Skills in label reading, attitudes about diet & health, daily fat intake	T ↓ fat intake, fried food & calories; ↑ label reading skills at follow-up compared to control	Supports peer leaders, & promise of skills training to reduce risks pre-diabetes

(continued)

Table 2.2 Interventions with diabetic adults *(continued)*

Author (year)	Objective	Design	Intervention	Mode	Sample	Outcome measures	Results	Notes
Bradshaw et al. (2007)	Evaluated resiliency training with adults	RCT 2-group pre-post, post-3 & 6 month follow up design; T & C(UC) groups	15 hour training with 10 modules	Small group	T = 30 C = 37	Glucose monitoring, daily diaries on eating & exercise, scales on self-efficacy, locus of control, social support	T ↑ improved psycho-social measures; no change in diet, glucose or activity compared to C(UC) group	
Forlani et al. (2006)	Evaluate an educational intervention based on empowerment	Non-random, 2-group pre- & post 12 month test design with a convenience sample; T = 54 C = 36 (refused to participate)	Eight 2-hour sessions on diabetes knowledge, diet, coping with diabetes, lifestyle changes, & seeking social support	Small group	T group average 43 y/o; 38% male; C group average 41 y/o; 66% male	Glucose monitoring SF-36, PGWB on anxiety, depression, well-being	T ↑ improved glucose control, SF-35 & anxiety, depression and well-being scores compared to C group	Limited by design & small sample
Gallegos et al. (2006)	Evaluate education + counseling intervention with adult men with Type 2 DM	RCT 2-group, repeated measures design; T & C (UC) groups	Combined intervention in 6 sessions (1.5 hr each) over 50 weeks on ethnic preferences & beliefs, diabetes management	Small group + individual sessions	T = 25 C = 20	Glycemic control, DM self care & adaptation to DM	↑ Glucose control & self-care at post-test points	

Author (Year)	Purpose	Design	Intervention	Format	Sample	Measures	Results	Conclusion
Gilliland et al. (2002)	Compare 2 family-centered interventions with Native American diabetics	Non-random 3-group, pre-post 12 months comparison design	10 sessions of culturally shaped education on diabetes management, & social support in MFG + single family sessions or single family sessions only	MFG & individual family sessions	All averaged 60 y/o T1=32; 72% female T2=39; 74% female, C=33; 91% female	Glucose levels & weight loss	↓ Glucose levels & ↑ weight loss in T1	Though with small sample, does give culturally adaptation methods on intervention & educational materials
Greaves et al. (2008)	Evaluate individual counseling with MI on behavioral changes with overweight adults	RCT 2-group comparison pre-post 6 month design; T=72; C=69; UC + information booklet only	Motivational interviewing to achieve behavioral changes for diabetic control	Individual	T=64% female; 53 y/o; C=64% female; 55 y/o	Glucose control, daily logs of activity	More of T group achieved glucose targets & ↑ physical activity compared to C group	MI shows promise in changing lifestyle behaviors for diabetic control
Smith et al. (1997)	Pilot study evaluating MI intervention + weight loss program with older diabetic women	RCT 2-group pre-post comparison design; T=combined intervention; C=weight management only	16 week weight management program + 3 MI sessions	Small group + individual sessions	41% African American; all women T=10 C=6	Food journal, glucose levels	T=glucose control at post-test compared & better journaling to C group	Very small sample, MI efficacy supported

(continued)

Table 2.2 Interventions with diabetic adults *(continued)*

Author (year)	Objective	Design	Intervention	Mode	Sample	Outcome measures	Results	Notes
Smith-West et al. (2007)	Evaluate revised weight program + MI with diabetics	RCT comparison 2-group, pre-post, post 6, 12, & 18 month design; T=42 group session +5 MI sessions; C=42 group session + 5 placebo sessions	18 month educational weight loss program + motivational on behavior changes for effective diabetic control program of 42 sessions	Small group + single sessions	T=109; 39% African American 47% married & ~54 y/o; C=108; 38% African American 38% married & ~52 y/o	Glucose & weight monitoring treatment adherence	T ↑ improved glucose control & weight loss at 6, 12, & 18 month post test	MI appears effective in changing diabetes management behaviors; good details of intervention & methodology
Vincent et al. (2007)	Evaluate a culturally tailored intervention with Mexican American Type 2 diabetics	RCT 2-group pre-post test & post 4 week design; T1 = intervention on the reservation C=UC at the clinic	Culturally tailored skills for living with chronic illness, diabetes knowledge & self-care; weight control	Small group	Sample 37–69 y/o; 71% women; T1=10 T2=7; no details of the 2 groups	Weight, BMI, glucose monitoring& physical activity; diabetes knowledge & self-efficacy; medication use	T = ↑ diabetes knowledge & self-efficacy, medication adherence & ↓ BMI compared to C group	Very small sample; details of cultural shaping of the intervention given

Notes: T = intervention/treatment group; T1 = 1st intervention group; T2 = 2nd intervention group; T3 = 3rd intervention group; C = control or comparison group; UC = usual care (e.g., physician visit, medication); ED = Emergency Department; MFG = multi-family group; DM = diabetes mellitus.

Overall, it is heartening that so many interventions have been studied with this population that are appropriate for social work practice, and have evidence of promise. Given the growing numbers of children and youth with diabetes it is also positive that school-based interventions have received attention in evaluation research. In sum, however, given the prevalence of Type 1 diabetes, more research is needed both in school settings and other settings as well.

In summary, the findings of the systematic review on evidence for interventions in this area suggest that practitioners have the opportunity to advance further evaluations in replicating the interventions and the designs of the studies discussed herein. Most notably the evidence supporting motivational interviewing with diabetics is supported as one-quarter of the total studies located in this systematic review evaluated its efficacy. This finding holds promise since both behavioral and cognitive change—the targets of MI—is requisite to effectively managing diabetes across the lifespan. In furthering the evidence supporting this intervention modality, the profession's quest for evidence-based practice could be further addressed.

Glossary

Beta cells—the insulin-producing cells in the pancreas.

Chronic illness—an illness characterized by the following: a serious, ongoing health condition that has a biological, anatomical, or physiologic basis and has lasted, or is expected to last, at least one year.

Co-morbid/co-morbidities—conditions or disease that are associated with a disease or disorder.

Diabetes—a metabolic disorder of the body that interrupts or prevents the body's ability to use glucose.

Etiology—a term that refers to the cause or causes of a disease or abnormal condition as well as the branch of medical science dealing with the causes and origin of diseases.

Glucose—the type of sugar derived from foods that moves into the bloodstream and provides fuel for the body's activities and growth.

Glycemic—a term relating to the term glucose, often used in relation to blood levels (i.e., glycemic level).

Hyperglycemic—having a higher than normal level of glucose in the blood.

Hypoglycemic—having a lower than normal level of glucose in the blood.

Insulin—the hormone produced in the beta cells of the pancreas.

Insulin-dependent—a type of diabetes that cannot be controlled through diet and activity, but must be controlled through the taking of insulin in either an oral or injectable form.

Ketoacidosis—a diabetic coma resulting from very high levels of sugar (glucose) in the blood.

Morbidity—any departure, subjective or objective, from a state of physical or psychological well being, may be expressed as a proportion of persons per 100,000 persons with a particular diagnosis or condition.

Mortality—the number of deaths in a given year per 100,000 persons in a defined population; the measure of the occurrence of death in a defined population during a specified interval of time.

Non-insulin-dependent—the type of diabetes that does not require either oral or injected insulin to maintain glucose control in the blood.

Pancreas—the organ in the body that produces insulin (in beta cells), and then releases the insulin into the body. The pancreas is located behind the stomach.

Prevalence—the proportion of a population having a disease, diagnosis, or medical condition over a specific period of time (e.g., year) expressed in a percentage.

Risk factor—an established direct cause of, or contributor to, the morbidity or mortality of a particular diagnosis or medical condition.

Sequela(ae)—an after effect of a disease, injury, procedure, or treatment.

A Scenario in Diabetes and Questions for Reflection and Discussion

Susan, a 15 year old, has Type 1 diabetes, diagnosed when she was 11 years of age. Susan is the youngest of three children with two older brothers, aged 17 (Nick) and 19 (Warren) years of age. She is currently in the ninth grade in a middle school; she should enter the community high school, located across the city, next year for her tenth grade. Both of her brothers attended the same middle school as Susan currently does. Susan's diabetes is generally well controlled with daily injections of insulin, and monitoring of blood glucose levels three times a day. Normally Susan manages each of these tasks on her own while at school. More recently, school personnel have become concerned, as she has reacted negatively when they asked about her completion of these diabetes management tasks. Her academic performance has never been a concern. What has at times concerned the school staff are her self-isolative behaviors among her peers. Recently the staff has observed that she has dressed differently. Susan's parents both have careers; her father is an officer in a local bank, and her mother is a landscape designer with her own company.

1) What are the possible developmental tasks with which Susan is contending? Does she appear to be "on time" with those tasks? How may her diabetes and its management influence her attainment of those developmental milestones?
2) What are the stressors and issues affecting her family and Susan's place in the family given the context of her diabetes?
3) How would you assist the school staff in their interactions with the family and in particular with Susan at this time? Should and, if so, in what ways staff connections to the high school to which she is to transfer for the tenth grade occur?
4) And, how would you revise your responses were Susan in the scenario to be in foster care because of medical neglect? How might that affect your:

   a) recommendations to school personnel?
   b) decision to contact the family, in this case the foster family, or not?
   c) decision to involve her brothers, or not?

5) What intervention or interventions would you select for work with Susan and/or her family in the original scenario and in its revisions (i.e., #4 above)?
6) How would your reflections to the above questions change were Susan a male, aged 43 with Type 2 diabetes?

3   Hypertension

- ♦ Who is affected by hypertension?
- ♦ What is hypertension? What are the treatments and medical regimens for hypertension?
- ♦ What are the psychosocial stressors associated with hypertension?
- ♦ What interventions are promising for social work implementation?
- ♦ Glossary
- ♦ Scenario

Introduction

Hypertension is the leading cause of cardiac disease, and cardiac disease is the leading cause of death in America. Hypertension, or high blood pressure, disproportionately affects minority and vulnerable populations. While the latter is not unique among health conditions, the extent of co-morbidities and sequelae of hypertension are grave, can result in disability, and are potentially life threatening. Hypertension is described as a major disease as evidenced by reports stating that one in every four Americans has high blood pressure (McCraty, Atkinson, & Tomasino, 2003; Wyatt et al., 2008). Most unfortunately, many, many individuals with high blood pressure do not know they have the condition, and, thus, the disease is untreated and uncontrolled. As listed by McCraty et al. (2003), the risk factors, and sequelae of hypertension are serious health conditions in themselves, and include heart attacks, strokes, kidney disease, and cognitive impairments including memory loss and damage to healthy brain tissue. The condition is disproportionately prevalent among at-risk and minority populations. It would appear that just within these few characteristics, hypertension qualifies as an area for social work commitments to providing the best practices available particularly with at-risk and vulnerable client populations.

Thus, this chapter first discusses the background issues, prevalence, and psychosocial stressors related to hypertension, the nature of the condition, medical treatments, and regimens. The chapter then discusses the eight interventions with promise of efficacy located in the systematic review of the present research. An exploration of the implications for practice, and future research, a glossary of relevant terms, and a scenario for discussion conclude the chapter.

Who is Affected by Hypertension?

For the period 2001 to 2004, high blood pressure affected an estimated one-quarter of Americans between 20 and 70 years of age, or more than 65 million adults (Borrelli, 2009; Centers for Disease Control & Prevention, 2006a). Overall, the Centers for Disease Control & Prevention report that high blood pressure affects slightly more women (26 percent) than men (24 percent) (2005a).

The rate of hypertension also increases with age across the lifespan. As a case in point, while in the 40 to 54 years old group, slightly less than one-third of men (30 percent) and one-third of women (33 percent) have hypertension, in those over 75 years of age, over two-thirds of men and over four-fifths of women have hypertension (Centers for Disease Control & Prevention, 2006a).

The scope of disparities in hypertension for African Americans is extensive. First, the prevalence of hypertension among African Americans is higher and more disproportionate than among any other racial group in the U.S. (Centers for Disease Control & Prevention, 2005a). The prevalence among African American men (38 percent) and women (40.5 percent) is higher than among white women and men (23 percent and 23.5 percent, respectively) (Lesley, 2007). Hypertension develops at earlier ages among African Americans, who are also more often diagnosed with extremely high blood pressure, and co-morbid serious sequelae (Lesley, 2007). As in illustration of the latter, African Americans with hypertension develop cardiovascular and kidney disease at higher rates than other population groups with hypertension (Lesley, 2007).

Littrell (2008) and Brummett et al. (2005) argue that the disparities by race for hypertension may be in part related to socio-economic disparities in the U.S. That is, the differences in prevalence of hypertension between the economically poor and the economically well to do in the U.S. may be linked to the enduring stressor associated with poverty, rather than just the economics of poverty. Research findings in other areas of health substantiate the linkages between poverty, race, and health status (Brummett et al., 2005; LaViest, 1993; Rich-Edwards & Grizzard, 2005).

Research estimating the total cost of care for hypertension in the U.S. uses various methodologies resulting in estimates ranging from 15 to 60 billion dollars annually. In analyzing the incremental cost of health care for high blood pressure more precisely, Balu and Thomas (2006) implemented probability sampling of a combined database of three national health care claims databases; sampling included only ambulatory, non-institutionalized adults 18 years of age or older with medically diagnosed hypertension, and prescribed anti-hypertensive medications. Incremental cost analysis uses costs solely attributable to the specific disease.

Balu and Thomas report that the total expenditures for the direct, non-hospitalization care of hypertension (i.e., physician visits, outpatient clinic visits, medications, emergency department visits) was more than 54 billion dollars nationally for the year 2001. They also estimate that the direct cost per hypertensive individual in their study was on average 1,100 dollars for the year. As the authors note, these findings are limited by the possibility of errors in the original diagnostic coding of the patients.

What is Hypertension?

Hypertension—the "silent" disease—is so named because the individual with high blood pressure may be unaware that they have the disease unless and until a health professional measures their blood pressure or severe outcomes occur, such as a stroke. Hypertension is a condition of having an elevated blood pressure or taking anti-hypertensive medication to control blood pressure (Wyatt et al., 2008). Blood pressure numbers are measurements of the force (pressure) of the blood on the walls of the arteries; arteries carry oxygenated blood from the heart throughout the body.

Hypertension or high blood pressure is classified as either "essential (primary)" hypertension or "secondary" hypertension. The complete cause of essential hypertension remains unclear, though it is generally believed to include genetics—as suggested by the role of a family history of the disease—in combination with lifestyle (Borrelli, 2009). Primary hypertension is the most common type of the disorder. Risk factor components for primary hypertension include:

- smoking,
- obesity,
- very limited or absence of physical activity,
- high levels of salt in the diet,
- genetics,
- family history of hypertension,
- consumption of more than one or two alcoholic drinks per day,
- stress,
- being of an older age.

The etiology of secondary hypertension, on the other hand, is much more complex. Secondary high blood pressure in contrast to primary hypertension is not only less common, but also is the result of another disease, thus the hypertension is *secondary* to a primary disease. Among the diseases to which hypertension is secondary are:

- disorders of the adrenal glands,
- kidney disease,

- some medications (e.g., corticosteroids, non-steroidal anti-inflammatory and decongestant medications, birth control pills),
- sleep apnea,
- birth defects in the aorta,
- pre-eclampsia (i.e., a condition related to pregnancy),
- Thyroid or parathyroid conditions.

The adrenal glands are located above the kidneys that secrete hormones (e.g., adrenalin). Disorders of the adrenal glands to which high blood pressure is secondary are caused by a disorder in hormone production of the adrenals, including:

- Cushing's syndrome (caused by too much cortisol secretion),
- hyper-aldosteronism (caused by too much aldosterone secretion),
- pheochromocytoma (a tumor that causes over secretion of hormones (e.g., adrenalin).

Kidney diseases that are causally related to secondary hypertension include, for example, tumors, kidney failure, and polycystic disease of the kidneys. Medications as noted above may cause secondary hypertension because of the actions of the medications themselves on arteries and/or on the kidneys. Sleep apnea is a condition wherein persons have episodes of not breathing while asleep. Pre-eclampsia is a condition occurring only during pregnancy and is resolved at or just after birth.

Hypertension is a serous disease identified as a risk factor for other major diseases as well. These include blockage of blood flow in the brain (i.e., a stroke), kidney disease or failure, heart attacks, coronary artery disease, retinopathy (blood vessel damage to the retina), and diabetes. Conversely, diabetes is a risk factor for hypertension, as are cardiac disease, and coronary artery disease.

Stages of Hypertension

Hypertension is diagnosed in either Stage 1 or Stage 2 as determined by the actual measurement of blood pressure. Blood pressure measurement includes two numbers (systolic and diastolic) with the former being the upper and the latter being the lower number (i.e., 120/80). Systolic blood pressure is the pressure of the blood during a beat of the heart; diastolic blood pressure is the pressure between the heartbeats. Normal blood pressure is equal to or less than 120 over 80. Elevated blood pressure sometimes referred to as pre-hypertension, means that when measured, the reading is on average 140 (systolic) over 90 (diastolic). Stage 1 hypertension is blood pressure measuring 140–159 over 90–99 and Stage 2 hypertension is blood pressure of 160 or higher, over 100 or higher.

Symptoms of hypertension are indicators of increased pressure within the cardiac system including coronary arteries and the heart itself. Generally, persons with undiagnosed high blood pressure experience one or more of the symptoms without knowing the reasons for the symptoms. Those taking anti-hypertensive medications (e.g., oral medications to control or reduce the level of blood pressure) may experience one or more symptoms when either under stress, neglecting a medication, and/or the medication needs to be adjusted by their physician. These symptoms include, for example:

- severe headache,
- mental confusion,
- tiredness,
- vision difficulties,
- chest pain,
- difficulties breathing,
- blood in the urine,
- palpitations or irregularities of heart rhythm.

What are The Treatments and Medical Regimens for Hypertension?

Though the medical regimen for treating hypertension has advanced with the recent development of effective pharmaceuticals, only about one-third of those with hypertension have control over their blood pressure (Bosworth, 2008; Chobanian et al., 2003). Pharmaceutical treatment of hypertension is medications that accomplish one or more of the following:

- dilate blood vessels,
- decrease certain chemicals that constrict blood vessels,
- help rid the body of water and salt through urinary excretion,
- slow the transfer of calcium into cells and widen blood vessels.

Dietary changes that help control high blood pressure control or limit the amounts and types of various foods associated with increases in blood pressure. One particularly well tested dietary program is the DASH (Dietary Approaches to Stop Hypertension) program. DASH is a structured eating plan that includes eating more fruits, vegetables, and low-fat products, including dairy products, reducing fat intake through limiting high fat foods, reducing red meats and sugary foods, increasing the amount of whole grain foods, and increasing foods containing potassium (bananas), and calcium (Lesley, 2007). The plan structures a specific number of servings per day of each of these categories of requirements, as for example, seven to eight servings of whole grain foods, and four to five servings of vegetables, and limiting the intake of meat and poultry to two or fewer servings. The DASH diet is reported to reduce blood pressure within a matter of a few weeks (Sacks et al., 2001).

The role of behavior in the control of high blood pressure receives consistent emphasis in the literature even though advances in pharmaceutical interventions have made significant advances in recent years. Of major concern is the role of adherence to medication, physical activity, and dietary medical regimens in controlling hypertension. Psychosocial and behavioral interventions to address adherence include strategies to modify eating patterns, activity patterns, medication use, smoking, and alcohol use, and stress management interventions, cognitive interventions, supportive interventions to reduce stress, and educational interventions.

What are the Psychosocial Stressors Associated with Hypertension?

The relationship between stress and health is complex and involves several systems. In terms of hypertension, the relationship of psychological stress and the response of the body's immune system, in particular its inflammatory response may be contributory to the development of hypertension. Though this pathway is unclear, it is suggested that the stress triggers the immune system, which in turn constricts blood vessels, and causes inflammation, which in turn prompts some hormones that control blood pressure, as well as contributing to weight gain and/or to higher cholesterol. Each of the latter is associated with scarring of the arteries (arteriosclerosis) and, thus with development of hypertension (Herbert & Cohen, 1993; Littrell, 2008). Littrell suggests that it is just that relationship of psychosocial stress and hypertension that substantiates the role of social workers intervening to enhance the effective management of hypertension.

Littrell (2008) discusses the stress related to the development of hypertension, particularly among populations with the highest prevalence rates of the disease. These factors include, most recently, work place stress due to the strain of high demand to get the work done, and the control of the worker in trying to get those tasks done is minimal. Work stress is also identified with situations where there is a mis-match or a discrepancy between the worker's effort and the rewards for working hard. The resultant strain is especially true and deleterious for competitive, hard-working persons in insecure employment situations where there is little recognition (Kivirmäki et al., 2005; McCraty et al., 2003). Research has recently demonstrated links between job strain and a narrowing of the arteries even when controlling for lifestyle behaviors and medical indicators that are risk factors for hypertension (e.g., smoking, alcohol consumption, exercise, cholesterol levels) (Hintsanen, et al., 2005).

One's environment beginning in childhood is a risk factor for poor health and certain health conditions, including hypertension. These environmental risk factors are poverty, lack of health care, obesity, and high-fat diets. These same characteristics are more common among racial minorities than they are among their white counterparts. Some research suggests that the experience of being a racial minority in a country with discriminatory and racist patterns in itself is deleterious to health (Aranda & Knight, 1997; Pinquart & Sorenson, 2005; Scarr, 1998; Sudha & Multran, 2001). The environment for racial minorities includes a greater likelihood of being unemployed—especially in the current global economic recession—of having a less extensive and less stable social support network, and the possibility of violent neighborhoods. In sum, the environment of racial and ethnic minorities can be termed a chronically stressed psychosocial context (LaViest, 1993). In relevance to the current discussion, and given the disparate prevalence rates for minorities, stress associated with being poor, and particularly chronic stress, suggests that stress is a logical target for intervention for those with hypertension.

Coping with stressful situations and stressful contexts in relation to minority populations receives attention in the literature. Some suggestions in the literature indicate that active participation in religious activities acts as a social support resource, especially in times of stress, and as a coping activity, particularly for minority populations (Brown, Garcia, Kouzekanani, & Hanis, 2002; Chadiha, Proctor, Morrow-Howell, Darkwa, & Dore, 1996; DeCoster, 2003; DeCoster & Cummings, 2004). In illustration, Brown, Garcia, et al.'s 2002 findings suggest that African Americans more frequently engage in prayer activities than other Americans do, and that doing so serves as a coping resource. Supportive mechanisms such as these may enhance non-adherence to medications and physical activity requirements to control hypertension (Morisky, Lees, Sharif, Liu, & Ward, 2002). Morisky and co-authors remind that non-adherence occurs in approximately one-half of persons diagnosed with hypertension and suggests that non-adherence may be related to lower socio-economic and educational status, and/or to specific characteristics and beliefs of cultural and ethnic groups.

Drevenhorn, Kjellgren, and Bengsten (2007), reflecting on a Cochrane review of evidence-based medicine on counseling for lifestyle change to reduce risk factors for hypertension, support the utility of changes in lifestyle on controlling hypertension. Also behavioral lifestyle interventions to reduce blood pressures is endorsed by Linden and Moseley (2006) who states that consideration should be given to psychological interventions as a first choice intervention, over medication alone that is, when the following are involved:

- The side effects of anti-hypertensive medications are severe.
- Lifestyle changes are inadequate in lowering blood pressure.
- Psychosocial support is needed to implement lifestyle changes.
- The hypertensive person would rather use non-drug interventions.
- When a family history, but no current indication of hypertension, indicates the wisdom of preventive measures.

In brief, the psychosocial stressors associated with hypertension are lifestyle challenges from the psychosocial environment, such as poverty, non-nurturing environments, work-place strains, and life events. The link between these stressors and hypertension is physiological. That is, the stress response path in the body stimulates the secretion of hormones and chemicals that in general constrict the blood vessels, and/or increase heart rates. These endpoints of the stress response result in increases in blood pressure, which in normal "flight or fight" response situations return to normal quickly when the situation is resolved. In the case of hypertension, however, the responses persist sustaining higher than optimal levels of blood pressure. As a result, while the advances in developing effective anti-hypertensive medications continue, daily routine and behavioral changes are also necessary for effectively treating hypertension. The promising interventions located in the present systematic review to accomplish behavioral and lifestyle changes are discussed below.

Promising Interventions for Social Work Implementation

The systematic review upon which this text is based located eight interventions evidencing promise of effectiveness and appropriateness for social worker implementation in practice with clients with hypertension. These studies implement the following modalities:

- small group work,
- small group work plus one-on-one individual sessions,
- one-on-one sessions.

Venues for the delivery of these modalities included clinic settings, home visits, and telephone conversations. Three of these interventions incorporated motivational interviewing techniques.

The efficacy of behavioral and educational interventions on controlling blood pressure was supported by the findings of an RCT study by Bosworth et al. (2008). The study's participants, in two primary care clinics, received the behavioral intervention (n = 319) or usual care (n = 317) over a two-year period (full sample average age 60 years and 47 percent African American). Participants had hypertension and a history of difficulty in adhering to their medical regimens, especially medications. The goal of the intervention was to change behaviors in order to enhance adherence.

The behavioral intervention's conceptual base combines the model of health decision making with targeted behavioral interventions, and the concepts of sequential changes in behavior from the transtheoretical model. The transtheoretical model incorporates elements of cognitive behavioral change in its emphasis on analyzing the advantages and disadvantages of a behavior change, enhancing self-efficacy, and reducing barriers to the behavior change.

The behavioral intervention was delivered via individual telephone counseling sessions implemented every other month with the participants on modules targeting knowledge about hypertension and medications, support from health providers and social relationships, diet regimen adherence, exercise, and reducing alcohol and smoking use as shaped directly by the participant's own issues, regimen and needs identified in initial assessments. The intervention included behavioral, problem solving, and motivational interviewing techniques. The authors report that early findings suggest that the treatment group had improved adherence to medication use, reduced anxiety and reduced depression levels compared to the control group during the first six months of the program. The intervention modules are extensively detailed in the article, including examples of conversations between the worker and a client, the latter facilitating replication of this low-cost, but apparently promising intervention.

Stewart and Davis (2003) also evaluated telephone delivery of one component of an intervention with the goal of modifying behavior in a randomized comparative group pre-post designed study. Participants were randomly assigned to the intervention group (n = 41) or to a comparison group (n = 42). Participants could choose one family member to participate in the study with them. The intervention began with an educational component plus a home-based exercise activity for all participants. The intervention group received in addition a telephonic intervention with the client and the chosen family member over the course of 24 weeks. The educational small group program occurred in a hypertension clinic of a hospital in conjunction with clients' medical appointments. Education involved hypertension knowledge and management, and risk factor modification discussions with printed materials, and an exercise plan to be completed at home. The follow up telephone sessions occurred twice each month—one with the client and one with the family member. Data was collected at baseline and after the conclusion of the study on hypertension knowledge and management (diet, use of salt, smoking, taking medications), exercise, symptoms of hypertension, and blood pressure. Results indicated that those in the intervention group adhered to medication regimens better, had significantly fewer symptoms of hypertension, were significantly more active, and more knowledgeable about high blood pressure than those in the control group were. Blood pressure levels of the intervention group were lower than, but not statistically different than those in the control group. The researchers suggest that the inclusion of family members created a support system for the clients, thus assisting in the modification of the clients' behaviors, and that changes in behaviors will over time reduce and/or stabilize blood pressure levels.

McHugh and colleagues (2001) implemented a home-based intervention with clients awaiting a coronary bypass in a pre- and post-intervention study over a period of 15 months. Participants were consecutively recruited in a major hospital-based cardiac clinic in Scotland and randomly assigned to either the intervention group (n = 49) or a control/usual care group (n = 49). The structured intervention was delivered to each participant's home each month, utilizing health education and motivational interviewing strategies. Outcome measures of the study included weight, physical activity levels, anxiety and depression scales, blood pressure control, and smoking. Measurements at the post-intervention time showed that overall health status as measured by the SF-36, and blood pressure improved significantly, while both anxiety and depression levels improved in the intervention group compared to control.

In response to the research linking work stress to blood pressure mentioned previously in this chapter, McCraty et al. (2003) evaluated a work-based stress management intervention in a randomly assigned intervention (n = 18) and wait-list control (n = 14) group, pre-test and post-three-month designed study on blood pressure, and levels of stress. Participants were required to have a physician diagnosis of hypertension. The intervention was a 16-hour program targeting hypertension through emotional re-focusing and restructuring with both learning and practicing the techniques; the study included heart rate feedback so that participants in the intervention could self-monitor and adjust accordingly. The intervention was a one day (eight hours) and two one-half day sessions delivered over a two week period where participants learned how to refocus emotions positively, and restructure the way they felt about work-related stressors, and included techniques to practice in the workplace on effectively and clearly communicating, and creativity in productivity.

Outcome measures included blood pressures taken three times before each session; and two psychosocial scales were completed at baseline and post-three-months. These were a scale measuring emotional and psychosocial health and work-related items and the Brief Symptom Inventory, measuring psychological distress. At post-test, the intervention group's blood pressure measurements had decreased significantly in both diastolic and systolic measures, and the group had significantly improved BSI scores compared with the control group. The authors provide extensive details of the intervention and the design of the evaluation study situated and referencing the workplace, its stressors, and effective mechanisms for reducing that stress. While the statistical significance is constrained by the small sample size, the clinical significance is considerable in light of the actual reductions in blood pressure measures of the intervention group (10.6 mm Hg systolic and 6.3 diastolic mm Hg). The utility of this promising educational and behavioral intervention rests in the detailed intervention and measurements, and that it addresses a population and a setting of import in the prevalence of hypertension. Given these factors, practitioners should consider replicating the intervention and its evaluation.

Intervening through psycho-educational and behavioral small groups on workplace stress as indicated by blood pressure was also evaluated in a RCT evaluation of an eight-week intervention (Nickel, Tanca, Kolowos, Pedvosa-Gil, & Bachler, 2007). Participants were recruited through advertisements, and screened for levels of stress overall, and specifically work-stress, and hypertension in initial phone interviews. The participants who met the study's criteria were randomly assigned to either the intervention (n = 36) or control group (n = 36). Participants were male, and ranged in age from 18 to 60 years. Participants completed daily blood pressure measurements through the eight-week research period, salivary cortisol levels several times per day, and three pencil and paper instruments on chronic stress, the State-Trait Anger Expression Inventory (STAXI), and the SF-36, measuring health-related quality of life, prior to initiation of the intervention and after its completion. Cortisol is an adrenal hormone that is excreted in increased amounts in response to bio-psycho-social stressors.

The small group intervention included components on the nature of stress both psychologically and physiologically, effects of coping on stress and coping strategies. Results indicated that the intervention group had significantly reduced blood pressure, and levels of each of the scales compared to the control group. While limited in its generalizability, the findings of this study is supportive of small group work with hypertensive men of a mixture of ages and to move the intervention on stress into a setting reported to be the source of stress overall and in the specific to the stress related to hypertension. Thus, the sample size and possible bias is a concern, the research the modality of the intervention. Last, this study creatively incorporated both medical and psychosocial outcome measures linking the health condition under study to both.

The efficacy of a combined behavioral combined with an established dietary change intervention program (DASH) on controlling blood pressure was supported in a randomized controlled study examining the effectiveness of lifestyle-educational intervention on hypertension in four clinics through a three-group pre-test, repeated post-intervention measurement design (Appel et al., 2003). Participants who had above optimal blood pressures, were not adhering to antihypertensive regimens medications, and did not have co-morbidities were randomly assigned to two intervention groups or a control group. Approximately two-thirds of each group were women, and one-third were African American, and low literacy levels. The treatment groups involved small group educational sessions (14 sessions) plus four one-on-one counseling sessions. The educational component of the T1 intervention (n = 268) was small group education on limiting salt and alcohol, and increasing physical activity; the T2 intervention (n = 269) was the small group educational group identical to that in the first treatment group plus the DASH diet. Both treatment groups included four individual counseling sessions. The control group received 30 minutes of advice in a single session only. Blood pressure monitoring over a six-month period showed that both educational interventions were effective in reducing and then maintaining blood pressure levels compared to only advice giving. The importance of these findings endorse the behavioral aspect of controlling hypertension, especially as the sample was hypertensives without medication in a randomized, controlled study and a large sample size.

The DASH dietary program was evaluated with African Americans in a major urban area at two community colleges; the design was a randomized, two-group comparison design (Lesley, 2007). Both conditions received the DASH program through interactive online programs; the intervention group also received the Problem Solving Training via online interactive media. The intervention group received the education program on the DASH plan combined with a social problem solving skills training (PST) on dietary problems and eating behaviors whereas the comparison group received only the DASH educational program. Participants, recruited at each college at informational desks by the researchers, were from 18 to 64 years of age, all were African American, excluding any who were on medically restricted diets, or had diabetes or kidney disease. The intervention group had 38 participants, and the control group had 40 participants; over two-thirds of the total participants were students and less than one-half had normal blood pressure.

The DASH educational program was computerized, including various official websites, such as that of the National Heart, Lung, and Blood Institute, pertinent to hypertension and in an online knowledge test that all participants viewed and completed, respectively. The problem solving intervention was also computerized and used interactive multimedia technology, and was viewed only by those in the intervention group. All participants completed their respective programs on laptops. The problem solving training program included questions created by each participant on eating habits with an open-ended answer format. Outcomes included the quality of the problem solutions identified given by participants during the intervention and at follow-up two weeks later in individual telephone interviews. Findings revealed that first, those in the intervention group had higher quality solutions during the intervention and at follow-up than those in the control group, and intriguingly, those with higher blood pressures whether formally diagnosed or not, had higher quality problem solutions overall. These findings lend support to both the problem solving skills training component, and suggest that those with hypertension are more receptive to knowledge about hypertension. The findings are constrained by the potential skew in the sample comprised primarily of students in their own academic environment. However, the details provided by the authors of each phase of the intervention are invaluable for replication, and the findings support the use of these multi-media interventions in community, school, and other settings.

A four-year longitudinal study implemented in the clinics of a county-wide medical center in a diverse and large metropolitan area in a RCT designed study evaluated the effectiveness of three interventions to control hypertension, promote lifestyle change, and adherence to hypertension regimes (Morisky et al., 2002). The study implemented pre-test, post-six, and post-12 month design in the community-based intervention (Community Hypertension Intervention Project). Participants (N = 1319) were recruited from the center's patients with a diagnosis of high blood pressure, who had difficulty in controlling their hypertension. Two-fifths of the full sample was male, and over three-quarters were African Americans (77 percent). The three-pronged evaluation randomly assigned participating patients to one of three intervention groups:

- health education in a single one-on-one counseling session (T1 = 328);
- appointment tracking and reminders (T2 = 330);
- home visitation (T3 = 328).

or to the control group (usual care) (n-330). The intervention in T1 was based on motivational interview techniques. Both T1 and T2 groups had significant decreases in blood pressure at the six, and 12 month post-intervention points. The findings on the T1 intervention modality support the value of educational interventions with this population, especially maintenance of lower blood pressure over a long-term period. Of interest is the finding that the home visitation intervention (T3) did not provide significant improvements in blood pressure control over the other two interventions, though many in the home visitation group did improve in that outcome. Given the rates of the disease and the higher rates of negative consequences, such as increased morbidity and mortality among inner-city, African Americans, these findings are of note for the replication of the intervention with promise of efficacy and for replication of the study's rigorous design. More importantly, it is a longitudinal study—very rare in an evaluation of intervention efficacy.

In brief, the interventions showing some promise of effectiveness discussed above include small group, and one-on-one modalities either alone or in combination, delivered in the workplace, at home, in colleges, and in clinic settings. Three of the interventions incorporated motivational interviewing (Bosworth et al., 2008; McHugh et al., 2001; Morisky et al., 2002) once again supporting MI for intervening in physical health conditions. (See Table 3.1 for summarizations of the promising interventions for hypertension discussed in this chapter).

Implications for Practice and Future Research

The interventions located in the present systematic review offer practitioners promising opportunities for effective practice with hypertensive clients in changing their lifestyles and behaviors to control their hypertension. Taken together the interventions were evaluated across several settings and specifically with the racial and age groups with the highest prevalence rates of the condition. This is encouraging and asks that social workers implement them, and further advance the state of interventions showing evidence in health care practice. The utility of motivational interviewing in three of the studies suggests that MI is a valuable approach in changing the behaviors necessary for control and management of high blood pressure. In sum, changing the behaviors and lifestyle attendant to effective control is crucial in deterring the grave life-changing and life-threatening co-morbidities and sequelae of hypertension. MI has attributes that make its use in health care powerful. These are, of course, its base of evidence in diseases and conditions, and importantly the nature of its short-term approach. Both characteristics meet the priorities of health care currently in place. Both attributes also endear its use by social work practitioners in the twenty-first century.

Table 3.1 Interventions in hypertension

Author (year)	Objective	Design	Intervention	Mode	Sample	Outcome measures	Results	Notes
Appel et al. (2003)	Evaluate the DASH behavioral intervention + MI on Stage 1 hyper-tension in 4 clinics	RCT 2-group design; T = DASH; C = advice only	T = DASH 14 sessions on dietary, lifestyle changes + 4 1:1 sessions of MI; C = 30 minutes advice only single group session + 4 1:1 advice only sessions	Small group + 1:1 individual sessions	T = 269; C = 273; average 50 years; 62% female; 34% African American; none on medication	Blood pressure; weight, sodium intake	T = ↓ blood pressure, weight & sodium intake across all post-tests compared to C group	Large sample & proven dietary intervention support addition of MI in Stage 1 clients
Bosworth et al. (2008)	Evaluate MI on BP via telephone with adults from 2 clinics	RCT, 2-group; pre-post design	T = 319; C = 317; T = MI twice monthly over 2 years; C = UC	1:1 sessions via phone	Averaged 60.5 years; 47% African American; majority 12th grade education or less	Self-report BP, weight, adherence to regimen	T = ↓ BP & adherence ↑ to diet and activity regimen at post-test compared to C group	Large sample, constrained by use of self-report; extensive details of intervention; supports MI

Author (year)	Purpose	Design	Intervention	Delivery	Sample	Measures	Findings	Comments
Lesley (2007)	Evaluate online DASH + problem solving training on BP & diet of urban African Americans	RCT 2-group comparison pre & multiple post test design; T=DASH + PST; C=DASH only	T=DASH + Problem Solving Training via online interactive program; C=DASH online only; setting community colleges	Individual via laptop computers	T=38; C=40; both 40% male; 18–60 years old; 2/3 college students	Quality of problem solving abilities in BP scenarios	T=↑ problem solving abilities compared to C group at post-test points	Supports the validity of DASH + PST & feasibility of community college laptop-based intervention
McCraty et al. (2003)	Evaluate work-place program on stress, & BP	RCT 2-group pre-post & post-3 month design in workplace; T=intervention; C=no intervention	T=16 hour health education of 1 full day & 2 half-day sessions	Small group	T=18, average age 48.2 years; C=14, average age 48.2 years; all male	BP; work stress scale & Brief Symptom Inventory	T=↓ BP, work stress & BSI levels; C=no changes	Very small sample; setting is unique in research on hypertension
McHugh et al. (2001)	Evaluate home delivered program to improve cardiac risk factors	RCT 2-group, waitlist controlled; T=intervention; C=UC waitlist	T=education on cardiac health + motivational interviewing	Individual home-delivered	T=62, 80% male, median age=63.0 years, C=49, 71% male, median age=61.1 years	SF-36, anxiety, depression, weight, physical activity, BP	T ↓ weight, anxiety, depression, & BP; ↑ improvement in health status & SF-36 scores compared to C group	Incorporates motivational interviewing in home-delivered intervention; small sample is limiting

(continued)

Table 3.1 Interventions in hypertension (continued)

Author (year)	Objective	Design	Intervention	Mode	Sample	Outcome measures	Results	Notes
Morisky et al. (2002)	Evaluate 3 interventions on lifestyle change & BP control with poorly controlled BP with inner city, diverse hypertensives	4-year, RCT 3-comparison & control group, pre-post 6 & 12 month design; T1 T2, T3 = interventions C = UC	T1 = health education (328); T2 = mailed reminder of appointments (330); T3 = home visit including family member (328); C = 330	1:1 sessions	40% male; 77% African American; 21% Hispanic; average age = 53.5 years; 80% or less had high school diploma	BP, BP regimen adherence	T1 ↓ & T2 ↓ BP sustained over 12 month period compared to T3 and to C groups	Emphasis on culturally salience of intervention & delivery; long-term design contributes to support of findings
Nickel et al. (2007)	Evaluate a small group psycho-education & behavioral intervention on workplace stress & BP	RCT 2-group, pre-post test design; T = intervention; C = UC	T = 8 weekly sessions of education on stress, coping & stress management	Small group	T = 36; C = 36; all male, aged 18–60 years	Daily BP & cortisol saliva test, STAXI, SF-36	T = sign BP ↓ & ↓ scores on each scale at post-test compared to C group	Details of each session provided; small sample & sampling bias are limiting

| Stewart & Davis (2003) | Evaluate an education + telephonic support intervention | RCT 2-group comparison, pre & post-test design; T1 & T2 | T1 = education + bi-weekly support via phone, including one family member; T2 = education only | Small group + individual phone sessions | T1 =41, average age = 56.3 years; 17% white; 76% unemployed; T2 =42, average age = 58.6 years; 69% unemployed | Weight, BP, adherence to BP regimen, BP knowledge, stress scale | T1 $\downarrow$ BP, $\downarrow$weight, $\downarrow$ stress scores & $\downarrow$ salt intake & $\uparrow$ BP knowledge at post-test compared to T2 | Innovative use of phone to deliver brief supportive counseling; small sample & lack of follow-up measures are limiting |

Notes: T = intervention/treatment group; T1 = 1st intervention group; T2 = 2nd intervention group; T3 = 3rd intervention group; C = control or comparison group; UC = usual care (e.g., physician visit, medication); MFG = multi-family group; BP = blood pressure reading.

Glossary

Atherosclerosis/arteriosclerosis—blood vessels can be visualized as tubes within which blood flows; these two terms are interchangeably used to identify a disease process of narrowing of that open space inside blood vessels.

Chronic illness—an illness characterized by the following: a serious, ongoing health condition that has a biological, anatomical, or physiological basis and has lasted, or is expected to last, at least one year.

Co-morbid/co-morbidity(ies)—conditions or disease that are associated with a disease or disorder.

Diastolic—the pressure measured between heartbeats.

Hypertension—high blood pressure; indicated when blood pressure frequently goes over 140/90 mm Hg (i.e., measured in millimeters [mm] of mercury [Hg]).

Hypotension—low blood pressure.

Incidence—the rate of an occurrence of a disease or disorder per a number of persons (i.e., 100,000 or 1,000).

Morbidity—any departure, subjective or objective, from a state of physical or psychological well being, may be expressed as a proportion of persons per 100,000 persons with a particular diagnosis or condition.

Mortality—the number of deaths in a given year per 100,000 persons in a defined population; the measure of the occurrence of death in a defined population during a specified interval of time.

Prevalence—the proportion of a population having a disease, diagnosis, or medical condition over a specific period of time (e.g., year) expressed in a percentage.

Primary hypertension—high blood pressure caused by a variety of factors, such as genetics, fat intake, weight, not due to another disease or disorder.

Risk factor—an established direct cause of, or contributor to, the morbidity or mortality of a particular diagnosis or medical condition.

Secondary hypertension—high blood pressure that is caused by a primary disease (e.g., kidney disease).

Sequela(ae)—an after effect of a disease, injury, procedure, or treatment.

Systolic—the blood pressure measured during heartbeats.

A Scenario in Hypertension and Questions for Reflection and Discussion

Dan Washington is a 34-year-old man, the branch manager of a large bank in the city, divorced, and the father of three children, two sons aged eight and 11, and one daughter aged 13. He has been divorced for about three years; his children visit him only occasionally, as his ex-wife is not particularly willing to share custody or parenting. Mr. Washington's diagnosis of primary hypertension was made a year and one-half ago; he has taken an oral medication once a day since that time. He has no other health conditions. During his most recent check up with his physician, he was instructed to begin monitoring his blood pressure daily and to contact the doctor if any pressure reading exceeded 155 over 99. His physician voiced concern about Mr. Washington's weight gain of 30 pounds since his appointment a year ago. Mr. Washington responded that his work had gotten very stressful, with the loss of several major clients and client companies, and being told to lay off three office staff. He added that he used to jog three or four times a week, but just hasn't had the energy in recent months. The physician suggested he contact you for assistance with his hypertension management and weight. In your initial meeting with Mr. Washington, he seems delighted to tell you about his college days when he played basketball and was "buff." He offers that his life has become "just about work," just like his father's. In response to your family system assessment questions, he reveals that his father died last year of a heart attack at the age of 59. He seems apologetic about his weight gain, saying that he has become a fast food junky in recent months.

1) a) What are the psychosocial stressors with which Dan is currently contending?
   b) And, how are these specifically related to his hypertension and weight gain?

2) a) What knowledge about hypertension, and its risk factors do you share with him?
   b) What would you share with Mr. Washington about the lifestyle changes needed to manage hypertension effectively?

3) a) What promising interventions for work with Mr. Washington would you select about lifestyle changes for hypertension?
   b) What is your rationale for that choice or choices of interventions?

4) How would your responses to each #1 and #2 of the above vary, or not, were Mr. Washington a woman with the same demographic characteristics, health conditions, and situation?

5) How would you incorporate culturally relevant information about hypertension and necessary lifestyle changes for its management if Dan were an African American or Hispanic?

4   Obesity

♦ Who is affected by obesity?
♦ What is obesity, overweight, and extreme obesity?
  What are the medical regimens and treatments for these
  conditions?
♦ What are the associated psychosocial stressors?
♦ What interventions are promising for social work
  implementation?
  • Children, youth and families
  • Adults
♦ Glossary
♦ Scenario

Introduction

Being overweight or obese receives ongoing attention in the literature and
the media as the prevalence rates and knowledge concerning the co-morbidities of excessive weight increase. One primary motivator for this
attention is the escalating rates of overweight and obesity among, not only
adults, but among children and adolescents (Levine, Ringham, Kalarchian,
Wisniewski, & Marcus, 2001). Understanding the psychosocial, economic,
and health complexity of these conditions is essential for practitioners to
effectively intervene. This chapter first discusses the prevalence rates,
relevant medical knowledge of the conditions and co-morbidities, medical
regimens and treatments, and the psychosocial stressors and sequelae
attendant to being overweight or obese for children and youth, and for
adults. Second, the 12 interventions promising efficacy located in this
systematic review are presented. The chapter concludes with an overview
of the implications for practice and future research, a glossary of related
terms, and a scenario with questions for reflection and discussion.

Who is Affected by Obesity and being Overweight?

The number of persons identified as overweight overall in America is
increasing dramatically. Current estimates are that 72 million adults are

overweight or obese (Ogden, Carroll, Curtin, McDowell, Tabak, & Flegal, 2006). According to the Centers for Disease Control & Prevention for the period of 2003–2004, nearly two-thirds of adults over the age of 20 in the U.S. were overweight and one-third of those were obese (Centers for Disease Control & Prevention, 2006c; Lang & Froelicher, 2006). The following comparison may facilitate understanding the remarkable increases in the prevalence rates of these conditions. That is, in 1990 no state had a prevalence rate of obesity greater than 15 percent, whereas in 2006 only four states had rates of less than 40 percent (Bean, Stewart, Olbrisch, 2008). At present, one in three American adults is obese, a rate that is more than double the rate in 1980 (Ogden et al., 2006).

The rapid increases in these rates for children and youth are particularly disturbing. As commented by Haynes and colleagues (2008) the rates of obesity among young children (six to 11 years old) from the late 1980s compared to the period of 2003 to 2004 more than doubled (i.e., seven to 19 percent). Some estimates suggest that approximately 20 percent of children 12 years of age and younger in America are either obese or overweight (Ogden, Flegal, Carroll, & Johnson, 2002). Just as striking is the increasing prevalence in the adolescent population (12–19 years of age) where the rate more than tripled (five to 17 percent) as of 2003–2004 (National Center for Health Statistics, 2006). Other reports suggest that one-third of American children and youth is overweight or at-risk of becoming obese, a tripling of the estimate in three decades (Centers for Disease Control & Prevention, 2006c; Bean et al., 2008).

The prevalence of obesity and risk for obesity in racial and ethnic groups, as true of other health conditions discussed in this text, is disproportionate across children, youth, and adults compared with their representation in the total population (Befort, Nollen, Ellerbeck, Sullivan, Thomas, & Ahluwalia, 2008; Ogden et al., 2006). For example, in regard to youth, the prevalence of those at-risk for being overweight among Mexican American and African American children and teens (37 percent and 35 percent, respectively), continues to remain higher than among their non-Hispanic white cohorts (33 percent) (Befort et al., 2008). As in illustration, the rates of extreme obesity among African American adults is more than double (10.5 percent) that of both non-Hispanic white (4.3 percent) and Mexican American (4.5 percent) adults. In terms of gender and race, African American women have higher prevalence rates of the conditions than their non-Hispanic white cohorts, and in comparison to some other ethnic and racial minorities (Befort et al., 2008; Ogden et al., 2006). Unfortunately, African American women's rates of related co-morbidities and of mortality are also higher than these rates for non-Hispanic white women of the same age (Befort et al., 2008; Fitzgibbon et al., 2008). Socio-economic level is also associated with obesity. As in illustration, Chang and colleagues indicate that lower SEC women have disproportionately high levels of obesity in comparison to women of higher SEC levels (Chang, Brown, Baumann, & Nitzke, 2008)

What Do The Terms Overweight, Obesity, and Extreme Obesity Mean?

Before explicating terms, it will be useful to appreciate what is known of the interactive nature of genetics in weight gain, and of being overweight or obese. A genetic component is now understood to play a role in both gaining weight and in the way and where fat is distributed in the body (Dreimane et al., 2007; Helmrath, Brandt, & Inge, 2006; Sogg & Gorman, 2008). As reported by Lang and Froelicher (2006), genetic inheritance may account for from one to two-fifths of the variance in individual body weight and in weight gain among individuals. Even as advances in investigating genes and genetic functions expand, it is likely that many genes (polygenic) interact to lead to being overweight. Dreimane and co-authors (2007) note that an estimated four-fifths of children born to overweight parents will become overweight either during childhood or later, while only 14 percent of children born to two non-overweight parents will do so. Regardless of genetic predisposition or genetic factors, other multiple behavioral aspects, such as consistent overeating, and inadequate physical activity, contribute to being overweight or obese. Moreover, as noted by Lang and Froelicher (2006) and by Helmrath et al. (2006), while multiple genes are involved, genetics interact with multiple environmental and psychsocial factors to contribute to obesity, rather than be determined by just genetics.

The terms "obesity" and "overweight" are commonly each used to characterize persons whose weight is perceived in America as above what is considered an "ideal" weight (Vallis et al., 2001). However, the standardized definitions of these terms come from medicine. As an example, the term "overweight" is operationalized as an adult weighing more for one's height as based on a standard chart of weight/height norms. The term "obesity" in adults is a more involved and multi-factorial construct. Obesity in adults is a condition as defined by the National Institutes of Health as having a body mass index (BMI), a weight-for-height scale, of 30 kg/height (NIH, 2000), and the extent of body fat places an individual at risk for several health problems (e.g., cardiac disease, hypertension). Accordingly, the National Institutes of Health's clinical guidelines for an obesity diagnosis in adults, developed from empirical evidence, requires an assessment including BMI, waist circumference, and risk factors for health conditions associated with obesity. Obesity is classified as one of two classes (I, II) and determined by BMI (I = 30–34.9; II = 35–39.9), the risk levels of associated diseases, and waist circumference.

A diagnosis of "extreme obesity" or "morbid obesity" means that the BMI (class III) is equal to or greater than 40.0, that disease risk factors and waist circumference are extremely high, and that the person is more than 200 percent, or 100 pounds over ideal weight for height (Choban, Jackson, Poplawski, & Bistolarides, 2002; Lang & Froelicher, 2006; Vallis et al. 2001). Further, morbid obesity is identified as a risk factor for serious health and medical consequences (e.g., cardiac and liver diseases and dysfunctions).

Do note that the designation of obesity and overweight status is different for children and youth from that of adults. These diagnoses are determined by percentile charts that identify weight by height and/or BMI per age (Haynes et al., 2008). Children who are at or above the ninety-fifth percentile for age are diagnosed as obese, while children between the eighty-fifth and ninety-fifth percentiles are identified as overweight.

The sequelae of being overweight or obese for health and for psychosocial well being are multiple and grave. As noted by Ogden et al. (2006) the following are sequelae for adults:

• cardiovascular disease,
• sleep apnea,
• hypertension,
• type 2 diabetes,
• stroke,
• chronic pain (largely due to joint or bone stress),
• postmenopausal breast cancer, and colon cancer,
• complications in pregnancy.

The co-morbidities of being overweight or obese for adolescents are similar, including, in addition, irregular menses and arthritis. Unfortunately, for those under 20 years of age who are overweight the likelihood that they will be obese in adulthood is more than twenty-fold compared with their non-overweight age peers (Haynes et al., 2008). Accordingly, the long-term medical sequelae for these teens are significantly grave.

The increasing prevalence of Americans who are overweight or obese has stimulated interest in analyzing the health care costs attendant to those conditions. Bachman (2007) analyzed the health care costs estimating that, compared to normal weight persons, expenditures for overweight and obese persons is from 21 percent to 111 percent greater. The range in cost is linked to the degree of obesity, with the greater costs related to those who are more obese. As an example, the increased expenditures for obese/overweight compared to normal weight persons are due to greater pharmaceutical expenditures for treating co-morbid conditions and sequelae (e.g., diabetes, cardiac disease). Specifically, the costs related to co-morbid conditions range from 77 to

227 percent greater compared to the same health care requirements of non-overweight persons. Bachman states that 9 percent of national health care costs relate to excess weight, with notable increases as the prevalence of obesity increases (2007). The financial cost of trying to lose weight through commercial weight-loss programs ranges from no cost to an estimated 2000 dollars (Vallis et al., 2001). Of course, success in these programs can lead to the prevention of medical co-morbidities, thus resulting in economic savings in addition to better health, decreased need for health care, and improved quality of life.

Vallis and co-authors found that over two-thirds of overweight and obese women in America report attempting to lose weight (2001). Tsai et al. (2009) found in their national telephone survey (n = 3500; African Americans = 10 percent, Hispanic = 16.5 percent, White = 73.5 percent) that African American and Hispanic adults are significantly more likely to use over-the-counter weight loss products and commercial weight-loss programs than are their Caucasian counterparts. Further, the researchers found that, across ethnic and racial groups, compared with lower SEC higher socio-economic status was associated with greater use of self-management, rather than commercial programs. Tsai and Wadden (2005) analyzed the effectiveness of three commercial weight-loss programs in the U.S. They report that there is minimal empirical evidence for efficacy of the programs, perhaps due to the absence of random controlled studies, or to the frequency of non-completion of programs. In recent years, pharmaceuticals for weight loss have become available. The empirical evidence on these oral medications suggests that they are effective, but note the necessity of behavior change in order for weight loss to be maintained (Egger, 2008; Latner, Wilson, Stunkard, & Jackson, 2002).

The use of surgical interventions for weight loss (bariatric surgery) for those who are morbidly obese is becoming more frequent for several reasons (Encinosa, Bernard, Steiner, & Chen, 2005). These reasons are:

- improved surgical techniques,
- poor rates of achieving weight loss through behavioral interventions and prescriptions,
- goals to deter or reduce the impact of the co-morbid conditions associated with extreme obesity.

The incidence of bariatric surgeries just between 1998 and 2002 increased more than five fold from six to nearly 33 per 100,000 adults (Nguyen et al., 2005; Santry, Gillen, & Lauderdale, 2005). Recently, the frequency of bariatric surgery for morbidly obese adolescents is also increasing with that rate tripling from 2000 to 2003. While that increase is quite dramatic, the actual total number of weight loss surgeries performed on teens is very small (i.e., 771 in 2003) (Tsai, Inge, & Burd, 2007).

Surgical weight-loss is expensive, and its cost is increasing; the cost increased by 13 percent in the years from 1998 to 2002 (Bachman, 2007).

The costs vary depending on the extent of pre-operative testing required (e.g., cardiac, sleep, esophageal studies), and post-operative hospitalizations for complications. Though weight loss surgery is financially costly, the long-term savings at present are unclear. However, these costs are likely to be no greater in the long run for morbidly obese individuals than non-surgical interventions to lose weight (Vallis et al., 2001).

Bariatric surgery causes weight loss because it either drastically reduces the amount of food that can be consumed by surgically reducing the size of the stomach, by disrupting the absorption of nutrients, or restricting food intake and interrupting absorption. It should be clear that the surgery does not "cure" obesity. Rather, the surgery changes the body's ability to consume and use food. The types of bariatric surgery include:

- restrictive procedures:

  - gastric banding
  - vertical banded gastroplasty (VBG)

- malabsorptive procedures:

  - intestinal bypass

- restrictive + malabsorptive procures:

  - Roux-en-Y

Restrictive procedures aim at producing satisfaction (feeling full) by abbreviating the size of the stomach. Malabsorptive procedures reconfigure connections between, or bypass section(s) of the small intestines, or remove segments of the small intestine altogether to reduce the body's absorption of food—thus, no matter how much is consumed, comparatively little is absorbed. The resultant limited absorption requires that the body use sources other than food for energy (e.g., body fat). The combination approach—the Roux-en-Y procedure—commonly referred to as the "lapband" procedure—both reconfigures the connections between the stomach and intestinal tract and reduces the size of the stomach to a small pouch. Among all weight-loss surgeries, the Roux-en-Y procedure comprises the vast majority of bariatric surgeries performed (Nguyen et al., 2005). For more in depth details of the anatomic aspects of each type of surgery than is relevant to the current discussion, the reader is referred to an article by Choban et al. that includes visual representations of each procedure (2002).

Findings evaluating the long-term outcomes of bariatric surgeries on weight loss are mixed. For example, evaluating the long-term outcomes of vertical banded gastroplasty (VBG), van Hout, Fortuin, Pelle, and Guus (2008) studied 91 VBG patients (pre-operative demographics: 87.5 percent female; average 38 years; 91.3 percent morbidly obese) over three years. Measurements of relevance to this discussion included weight loss, BMI, the SF-20 scale on psychosocial functioning, and the Dutch Personality Questionaire (NVP). At two-years post-surgery only 12 percent of the sample were still morbidly obese, and many had improved psychosocial outcomes. However, after the two-year point, no further improvements were found, and some deteriorated. As suggested by these authors, and others (Burgmer, Petersen, Burgmer, Zwaan, Wolf, & Herpertz, 2007), positive outcomes may be either short duration, or diminish progressively over time. Van Hout et al. (2008) report that approximately one-quarter of the patients in their study did not lose weight after surgery, and initial improved psychosocial improvements did not last. The authors attribute these less than optimal outcomes to non-adherence to dietary and behavioral regimes after VBG. In contrast, Wadden et al. (2007) in reviewing studies on the outcomes of bariatric surgery indicate expected weight loss and improved psychosocial outcomes, and similarly attribute failures to patients' non-compliance to post-operative plans.

Even in the best-case situations, the post-operative plan requires behavioral changes that are extensive. The plans include daily vitamin and mineral supplements, multiple changes in the types, amounts, and timing of foods consumed, frequent, but very small meals, and maintaining physical activity. Typical side effects of the surgery include recurrent or chronic diarrhea, nausea, and/or vomiting. When body chemistry becomes imbalanced from not adhering to vitamin and mineral supplement requirements, fatigue, headaches, and/or shakiness can occur. The behavioral changes that diet, medication regimes, and the psychosocial adaptation require are challenging and stressful, and often require professional guidance and intervention.

In summation, the escalating prevalence rates of obesity across all ages are startling, and worrying. The racial, ethnic, and socio-economic disparities of obesity overall have particular relevance for social work practitioners. The research extant suggests that there is likely no silver bullet available at present to resolve weight problems quickly and permanently. Rather, as being overweight and obese is a complexity of interacting factors, interventions need to include the bio-psycho-social context and issues. The following discussion on the related stressors is intended to provide that psychosocial context for practitioners.

What Are Associated Psychosocial Stressors?

The psychosocial, psychological, and emotional issues for individuals, who are overweight in a society that identifies being thin, and largely very thin for that matter, as ideal are multiple (Bean et al., 2008; Melcher & Bostwick, 1998; Vallis et al., 2001). As illustrated by Vallis and co-authors, and others, negative aspersions about overweight persons are frequent and may begin in early childhood, supporting the societal belief that overweight persons are responsible for their own obesity (Melcher

& Bostwick, 1998). Not surprisingly, given the negative attributions, and discriminating and stigmatizing beliefs coming from family members, colleagues, and friends, the psychological and emotional co-morbidities of obesity include: depression, negative self-views, and low self-esteem, in addition to social isolation, and difficulties forming and maintaining personal relationships (Bean et al., 2008; Sogg & Gorman, 2008; van Hout, Boekestein, Fortuin, Pelle, & van Heck, 2006). Evidence to date suggests that depression and being overweight or obese are related, with one-third higher rates of depression among overweight/obese women compared to their non-overweight peers; the findings comparing women and men suggest the relationship between weight and depression exists for women, but not men (Bean et al., 2008; van Hout et al., 2006).

For the morbidly obese, the negative outcomes of anxiety, poor body image, and social isolation are even more intense. That intensity is reflected in the findings of Kalarchian et al. (2007) of DSM Axis I diagnoses among 288 morbidly obese patients (83 percent female; 88 percent white) seeking bariatric surgery. Kalarchian and co-authors report that two-fifths of the women reported a major depressive disorder, and over two-thirds reported anxiety disorders. Possibly linked to these psychiatric disorders is the evidence that the negative reactions and beliefs of others about being overweight begins in early childhood, particularly for overweight or obese girls (Bean et al., 2008).

Some suggest that perceptions about weight and losing weight may be related to racial background. In a recent study of African American and white women, Chang et al. (2008) examined these constructs in a sample of women, including those who were of normal weight and those who were overweight, comprised of 200 African American and 201 white women (aged 18 to 50 years) in WIC centers. Measures by self-report included demographics (i.e., education level, age, racial group), dietary details (fat and caloric intake, eating patterns (at home or elsewhere), self-efficacy in dietary management and controlling eating patterns, emotional states associated with actually eating, and the frequency of fat-intake control behaviors. Not unexpectedly, fat intake predicted weight in both white and African American women. But more notably, rather than race independently affecting the measurement outcomes, educational level predicted weight management knowledge, weight management, and fat intake reduction. Variances between black and white women involved only specific domains within the construct of self-efficacy in managing one's weight. As emphasized by Chang et al., interventions to effect weight loss should be tailored in light of specific aspects of the targeted populations, rather than more globally.

The stressors for overweight/obese children and adolescents may be particularly acute as they simultaneously move through normative developmental stages and tasks. The psychological stress for children of being overweight/obese, according to Dreimane and co-authors (2007) and

Haynes et al. (2008), are poor body image and self-esteem, and feeling shameful, as well as related co-morbidities (e.g., diabetes, high cholesterol levels, hypertension, bone malformation).

In light of the developmental tasks of adolescence, the potential that obese and overweight teens may withdraw from social contacts, be unable to physically partake in some activities typical of teen life (e.g., sports, dancing) coupled with the importance of body image during this developmental period have psychosocial ramifications that cannot be overstated. For example, the developmental tasks of adolescence include forming relationships with peers, developing self- and gender-identity. Physical limitations as noted above can well deter activities that foster the achievement of the developmental tasks of adolescence. Haynes et al. (2008) include traumatic physical injuries among the negative consequences of obesity for adolescents due to physically being unable to use safety assurances, such as seat belts. Extreme (morbid) obesity among teens is associated with increased risk of suicide. Long-term negative psychosocial sequelae include, for example, suggestions that obese teens are less likely to marry, less likely to go to college, and more likely to be economically poor (Helmrath et al., 2006).

For those who undergo bariatric surgery, beyond the euphoria of expedited weight loss after years of attempts to do so, emotional challenges are also likely. These emotional challenges include changes in the ways the person is related to by friends and families, changes in their own body image and self-concept that may be difficult to inculcate, and unexpected reactions from others for who changes in the formerly morbidly obese person are challenging as well (Sogg & Gorman, 2008). The required adherence to post-operative regimens may be a struggle for adults, but may be especially troublesome for adolescent bariatric surgery patients (Sogg & Gorman, 2008).

In sum, the psychosocial stressors and potential negative sequelae of obesity across the lifespan are severe. In consideration of these stressors and sequelae, it is apparent that components of successful interventions should include content on self-efficacy, dietary patterns, attitudinal or perceptual views on dieting, body image, beliefs about ideal weight, motivation to change weight-related behaviors and coping with the stressors of weight loss and maintenance.

What Interventions Are Promising for Social Work Implementation?

Interventions Showing Promise of Efficacy with Children, Youth, and Their Families

Overall, there are 12 studies with promise of efficacy in intervening on obesity, overweight, and weight loss maintenance. One would have expected that interventions for overweight or obese children and youth would be readily available as their rates of obesity are growing so rapidly. However, only three studies evaluating interventions directly with children were located in this systematic review meeting current criteria. Fortunately, each of these studies has extensive details of the interventions, and of the evaluation design and methodology; one study includes motivational interviewing in its intervention package. These three studies are described below.

Yin, Wu, Liu, and Yu (2005) examined a multi-faceted intervention targeting weight reduction, improving knowledge, attitude and behavior related to weight loss among fourth-grade children overweight for their height (n = 118) in a pre-test, post-test with an intervention (n = 66) and control (n = 52) group, randomly assigned designed study. The small group intervention was based on interactive reciprocal conversations between educators and children tailored to each child's needs as indicated at baseline and shaped by feedback from the child as to the pace and content of each session. Those researchers found significantly improved knowledge, slightly but not significantly improved behaviors, and no changes in attitudes concerning weight, weight loss and diet in the intervention group. Of note is that the authors provide useful details of the intervention, including extensive examples of behavioral and reflective conversations between the child learner and the teacher leader.

A randomly assigned two-group comparison evaluation by Dreimane et al. (2007) evaluated the effectiveness of an intervention with seven to 17 year olds whose weight was at or above the eighty-fifth percentile in standardized charts. The pre-post design compared a six-week intervention to a 12-week intervention program with repeated measures located in a university hospital. Participants were referred from hospital clinics and physicians; 180 children and teens with their parents participated in the eight-week program and 84 in the 12-week program. In terms of weight control, measurements included weight, height, BMI, and the child health, emotional well being, self-esteem scale (CHQ) and family questionnaires. At least one parent attended the 90-minute sessions with their children; components included educational and behavioral interventions on exercise, nutrition, and family involvement strategies. Each session began with the children engaged in physical activities such as dancing, modified sports activities; during this segment, parents were involved in separate small groups covering obesity knowledge, and the importance of supporting children's efforts to lose weight. After completion of the two separate small group interventions, there was a nutritional education session and a behavioral modification session with both children and parents. Outcome measures were recorded by children and youth in daily dietary and exercise journals repeatedly throughout the eight and the 12-week programs; parents were required to verify these journals, and to complete a family cohesion scale and the CHQ at baseline and post-intervention. Analysis of the outcomes demonstrated that the children and parents in the eight-week program had significantly higher family cohesion scores, and these children and youth lost significantly more weight than those in the 12-week program. More importantly, those children who began with higher BMI scores (i.e., were more overweight) made significantly greater improvements than others in both intervention groups. Children and teens that lost more weight compared to those who lost less also had higher self-esteem and emotional well being scores at post-test. These findings are supportive of family involvement in intervening with childhood and adolescence obesity with possible economic cost savings for the more effective, but shorter intervention program. Of note, the article provides comprehensive details of the content of the sessions.

A study discussed in the chapter on diabetes (Channon et al., 2007) is also applicable to this discussion of obesity as well. The RCT study evaluated MI with 66 adolescents with Type 1 diabetes. For purposes of the present chapter, however, though the study's objective was not weight loss or weight maintenance, weight loss was included as an indirect indicator of glycemic control among the participants. The reader will recall that Channon and colleagues randomly assigned the participants to the intervention or to the control group (usual care) with baseline and post-six, 12 and 24 month measurement points. The intervention included individual motivational interviewing sessions over a one-year period, measuring glucose control, glucose monitoring, the use of insulin, weight loss, and psychosocial measurements. In addition to significantly reduced worries and anxiety scores, participants in the treatment group reported increased weight loss in comparison to the control group. Given the length of the study, it is supportive that weight loss was maintained through the 24-month study, indicating the efficacy of the intervention in terms of one of the major methodological challenges of evaluating interventions on weight loss and weight management.

These three intervention studies provide the details and innovations for practice with overweight/obese children and teens with small group and individual interventions. Of particular relevance to social work practice is that these studies include details for replicating the intervention. It is to be hoped that such replications can lead to additional evaluations of efficacy for intervening with overweight or obese children and adolescents, and their families.

Interventions Promising Efficacy with Adult Clients

Nine studies intervention evaluations were identified in the systematic review that promise efficacy with adult clients. Of these, three studies evaluated the effect of motivational interviewing on weight loss or weight loss maintenance with adults. It is beneficial that the application of MI to obesity and weight loss has been explored by Dorsten (2007). Dorsten discusses the applicability of motivational interviewing in weight loss interventions, and its potential for efficacy, noting some of the studies discussed below in this section of the current chapter. In brief, Dorsten identifies three elements of behavior change in MI:

1) increasing motivation;
2) enacting change activities;
3) using relapse prevention tactics.

Eliciting behavioral or situational factors that shape an individual's readiness for change—a standard component of MI—is essential in changing those behaviors that may work against losing weight. As Dorsten summarizes, the benefits to the client of losing weight and the client's ambivalence to change are equally essential in practice with overweight clients. With that brief overview of MI applied to weight loss, the following section of this chapter discusses the three MI studies located in the systematic review for efficacious interventions.

Carels and co-researchers (2007) examined the efficacy of motivational interviewing (MI) in a randomly assigned two-group comparison study of the effect of a weight-loss intervention with voluntary adult participants. Criteria for inclusion in the study were: being overweight (BMI >30), exercising less often than twice a week, being non-smokers, having clearance from their own physicians, and having no co-morbidities. The voluntary participants (n = 55) were matched on demographics, weight, diet and physical activity and then randomly assigned to a behavioral weight loss program with motivational interviewing (T1 = 28) or to the behavioral weight loss program only (T2 = 24). The 20-session (75 minutes each) behavioral intervention was based on previously implemented manualized curriculum (Carels et al., 2005). The curriculum targets increasing physical activity, and gradual weight loss, as well as improved diet. The MI intervention component delivered in individual sessions was designed to decrease ambivalence toward behaviors to lose weight. Findings suggest that the MI component significantly increased weight loss, and increased physical activity more than the weight loss program alone. These findings are limited, of course, given the small sample size, but support the growing evidence for motivational interviewing in a number of health disorders. Notably the authors provide discussion and analysis of treatment integrity of the MI intervention through two clinical raters and a validated MI integrity scale and coding scheme.

Also supportive of the efficacy of motivational interviewing on the eating behaviors of adults associated with weight loss and weight management is a study by Resnicow et al. (2001). The study examined

MI intervention's effect on fruit and vegetable consumption, rather than carbohydrate or fat consumption, in a baseline and one-year follow up design implemented in 14 African American churches. The researchers conceptualized the target of increasing consumption of fruits and vegetables as indicative of dietary behavior patterns that, were the intervention successful, would be associated with weight loss. Second, the researchers were intent on evaluating the interventions with a culturally salient design, and with an intervention (MI) with strongly suggested efficacy for behavior change. Participants were assigned randomly to one of three groups:

- culturally relevant self-help group plus one telephone call;
- culturally relevant self-help group plus one telephone call plus three MI counseling telephone calls;
- a comparison group that received printed diet information only.

The MI group demonstrated significantly greater dietary changes at follow-up. Though not including psychosocial outcomes, this study lends promise for the use of MI in weight loss and control interventions.

Smith-West and colleagues (2007), expanding the intervention of their earlier pilot study (1997) on the effect of motivational interviewing on glucose levels of diabetics, evaluated the efficacy of the intervention on weight loss in a random, comparison group, baseline and repeated measures design. A total of 217 overweight women participated; they averaged 54 years of age, just over one-third was African American, and just over two-thirds were employed (Smith et al., 1997; Smith-West et al., 2007). The expanded weight loss program (42-sessions) was combined with either five sessions of MI over 12 months (T1 = 109) or with five attention-placebo sessions of instruction on various topics of health relevant to women over 12 months (T2 = 108). Measurements after baseline occurred every six months thereafter recording weight and height, attendance in the weight management group, and self-report diaries on daily eating and exercise activities. Participants in both the T1 and T2 groups lost weight over the duration of the study. However, weight loss in the T1 group was significantly greater at each of the six-, 12-, and 18-month outcome measurement points compared with the T2 group. Findings of this study again support the efficacy of the MI intervention on weight loss, and of long term intervening to prompt and maintain weight loss. In addition, the authors provide extensive details of their methodology and of the interventions implemented.

Four interventions other than those using MI to achieve weight loss, and weight control with adult clients were located. A discussion of these is provided below; the studies included small group interventions and one-on-one interventions either alone or in combined approaches.

Agurs-Collins, Kumanyika, Have, and Adams-Campbell (1997) report the findings of a RCT, pre-post-intervention evaluation of a weight-loss-program intervention with 55–79-year-old African American women recruited from clinics and physician offices and implemented in the clinics of a large metropolitan hospital. The participants in the intervention group (T = 32) engaged in a 12-week small group intervention plus one individual counseling session plus six biweekly follow up sessions; the control group (C = 32) received only usual care in the clinic setting. The small group sessions (90 minutes) focused on nutritional education, exercise activities, while the individual session targeted specific challenges of the participant in maintaining dietary control and being physically active. Outcomes of significance for the current discussion were that the intervention group had significantly greater weight loss, increased exercise activity, and increased diet and weight loss knowledge compared to the control group. Though this early study is constrained by its small sample size, findings lend support to the efficacy of group interventions combined with individual sessions and responds to the need for evaluation of interventions with minority populations.

Byrne, Meerkin, Laukkanen, Ross, Fogelholm, and Hills (2006) studied the efficacy of a personalized weight management program (PWMP = 41) compared to standard care (SC = 33) on weight loss in a RCT pre-/post-intervention and follow-up design. Participants were recruited in an Australian metropolitan area via radio messages, and newspapers. Two-thirds of the intervention group were women, averaging 62 years of age. Both groups were given standard nutrition and exercise advice, while the PWMP intervention group additionally received written materials to design their own diet and activity plans. Outcome measures on body weight, body composition, waist size, and fitness analyzed at post-intervention points demonstrated that the intervention group had significant improvements in greater weight loss, reduced body fat and waist measurement over baseline assessments than the standard care group. The findings imply that interventions that target self-efficacy through, in this instant, self-monitoring and self-motivation strategies in weight loss programs are promising.

One study evaluated the effect of interventions on maintaining weight loss over the long term among obese women, aged 21 to 60 years, in a randomly assigned three-group pre-test, post-test, and follow up design (Perri, Nezu, McKelvey, Shermer, Renjilian, & Viegener, 2001). The interventions of interest were diet plus exercise interventions of three types:

- behavioral therapy (BT; n = 15);
- behavioral therapy plus relapse prevention therapy (RPT; n = 20);
- behavioral therapy plus problem solving therapy (PST; n = 23).

The initial BT condition for all participants was a five-month long cognitive behavioral weight loss intervention composed of 20 weekly (two-hour) sessions on dietary knowledge about weight management, such as goal setting and self-monitoring, in small groups of 11 to 14 participants. After completing the BT intervention, those randomly assigned to BT for the evaluation received no further intervention, but were assessed after six and 12 months. The other participants were randomly assigned to either the relapse prevention (RPT) or the problem solving therapy (PST) group.

Those in the RPT engaged in a year-long program of support and psychoeducation; the PST intervention included developing coping skills and problem solving strategies. Outcomes of the study included weight changes and weight management skills. Analysis of findings after the conclusion of the 18-month program demonstrated that the PST (problem solving intervention) resulted in a greater proportion of members losing weight over the course of the program than either of the other two groups. Thus, for the long-term management of weight loss, problem solving interventions appear to be more effective than either behavioral or relapse prevention therapies. It is of note that these interventions are appropriate for social work practitioners, and speak to the need not often evaluated empirically of interventions for long-term outcomes in the treatment of being overweight or obese.

Painot, Jotterand, Kammer, Fossati, and Golay (2001) evaluated the effect of a combined nutrition and cognitive behavior intervention (NCB; n = 25) compared to cognitive behavioral intervention alone (CB; n = 35) on binge eating in a randomly assigned, baseline and post-test design. Participants were all women, Caucasian, and, on average, 42 years of age. Each group participated in a 12-week (1.5 hours each) small group. The nutritional portion of the combined approach targeted analyzing the nutritional components (i.e., calories, fat in food). All participants completed daily food diaries, recorded daily weight, and several psychological measures at pre- and post-test points. Psychological outcome measures were the Eating Disorders Inventory, Hospital Anxiety Depression Scale, and the Beck Depression Inventory. Findings demonstrated that the combination approach resulted in significantly greater weight loss, and improved psychological outcomes. These findings are limited by the small sample size; however, they do suggest that a combination of nutritional knowledge and behavioral change is more effective than either approach alone.

Unfortunately, in spite of the dramatic increase in the numbers of bariatric surgery performed, and reported associated psychosocial problems, the vast majority of research concerning weight-loss surgery is based on the surgery itself being the intervention, and resultant weight loss the only outcome. Only two studies meeting the criteria of the present research were located. The discussion of these two studies follows.

Hildebrandt implemented a study over a decade ago (1998) on post-Roux-en-Y gastric bypass patients on the effect of attendance in a support group on weight loss in a retrospective design. She identifies, in brief, the components of a support group intervention as helping participants to be hopeful, providing information, and motivating group cohesiveness. Participants in the study were all post weight loss surgery (Roux-en-Y procedure) patients who completed a mailed questionnaire regarding their post-operative experiences, demographics, and whether or not they had attended the center's support groups for bariatric patients. Responses from 69 patients attended the support group after surgery. Comparisons of support group attenders and non-attenders showed that there was a trend for attenders to lose more weight than non-attenders, though non-significant. The finding suggests that participation in a support group is related to weight loss subsequent to the Roux-en-Y bariatric procedure. However, that implication is greatly constrained due to the lack of random assignment, the retrospective design, and limiting methodologies.

A second more recent evaluation of the effect of participation in a support group for post-weight loss surgery patients is a retrospective comparison group design (T = 200; C = 100). The participants were 89 percent women, 61 percent married, and 81 percent white (Welch, Wesolowski, Pieput, Kuhn, Romanelli, & Garb, 2008). The treatment group sample was post-surgery patients attending the support group; the comparison group was post-surgery patients attending the bariatric clinic for regular post-op care. The support group focused on the medical regimens of post-bariatric care and behaviors. Demographics, weight loss, and health questionnaires were collected including author-developed Bariatric Self-Management Questionnaire (on behavioral adherence to diet, supplements, and physical activity). The researchers report that the latter subscale on physical activity of the behavioral adherence scale was significantly related to weight loss. The utility of the finding is very hampered by the use of self-report of weight loss, the non-random and retrospective design, and selection bias.

The implications of these two limited evaluations, as noted by others (e.g., Burgmer et al., 2007; van Hout et al., 2008), are the import of psychosocial interventions, and long-term follow-up with weight loss surgery clients. This implication reflects the need after surgery to adapt behaviorally to the multiple-dimensions of the medical regimen, and to adjusting to the psychological and emotional challenges as discussed previously in this chapter. It must be noted that, given the promise of motivational interviewing delineated earlier in this chapter on weight loss, it is appropriate that MI be evaluated in terms of intervening on post-weight loss adults.

To summarize the evaluations of the nine interventions for adults discussed above, it is notable that in three of the studies motivational interviewing was the intervention evaluated. The findings of those three studies reinforce the applicability and efficacy of this approach to behavioral change demonstrated in other areas of health problems. In addition, the remaining evaluations small group interventions either alone or in combination with individual sessions were employed. And, importantly, given the prevalence of obesity and being overweight among minority populations, only three of these studies were implemented with diverse populations. Thus, professional social workers should most clearly implement the promising interventions located in the present research with diverse client groups and populations. Second, the dearth of effective psychosocial and behavioral interventions for those having had weight loss surgery is disturbing, especially so in light of the rapid expansion of the numbers of these surgeries performed, and the consistent findings that psychosocial post-surgery and long-term problems occur.

Implications for Practice and Future Research

Overall the interventions discussed in this chapter explore several that have some evidence of efficacy for intervening with clients and client systems challenged by being overweight or obese. That motivational interviewing showed promise of efficacy in intervening with these problems is not surprising, but is re-assuring. The promise of this intervention for clients who are obese or overweight in assisting them to lose weight and maintain weight loss suggests that further implementation and evaluation of MI with in this area, and specifically, with overweight or obese adolescents may be fruitful.

However, two specific areas need to be incorporated in further empirical evaluations for promise of interventions. One area is the evaluations of interventions focusing specifically on adults, children, and teens from diverse backgrounds, particularly those backgrounds that have disproportionately high prevalence rates. Second, what are also generally lacking are evaluations of interventions for long-term weight loss and weight maintenance, including those for bariatric surgery patients.

These two gaps for the advancement of promising interventions for social workers call for practitioners to respond in two ways. First, workers are exhorted to gain the requisite knowledge concerning the weight and obesity and the promising interventions for weight loss and maintenance available. Second, practitioners need to become knowledgeable about weight-loss surgery and replicate interventions showing promise. Just as important are the development, implementation, and evaluation of psychosocial and behavioral interventions to address long-term weight loss and wellness objectives after bariatric surgery, and evaluations of these interventions.

In addition, MI as an intervention in post-weight loss surgery may prove beneficial as the numbers of these operations increase, including its use with adolescents seeking to lose weight. In summary, the negative sequelae of both overweight status and of obesity, especially among children, youth, and minority populations, speak clearly to the professional requirement that practitioners provide best practices in work with these at-risk populations.

Table 4.1 Interventions in obesity

Author (year)	Objective	Design	Intervention	Mode	Sample	Outcome measures	Results	Notes
Agurs-Collins et al. (1997)	Evaluate weight loss program in urban clinic with African American women	RCT 2-group, pre-post design; T=intervention; C=UC	12-weekly (1½ hour sessions each) on nutrition, exercise; individual sessions on dietary control	Small group + 1 individual session + 6 follow-up group sessions	55–79 y/o African American women, ½ unemployed; T=32; averaged 62 years old; 53% married; C=32; averaged 61 years old; 41% married	Weight loss, activity, dietary adherence	T=significant ↓ weight loss, ↑ dietary adherence & knowledge, & physical activity over C	Limited by small sample; targets high-prevalence population
Byrne et al. (2006)	Evaluate personalized weight management program (PWMP) metro city	RCT 2-group pre-post design; T=PWMP; C=UC	PWMP is nutrition & exercise advice & written materials to design own plan	Small group	Sample 2/3 women averaging 62 years of age; T=41 C=33	Weight, BMI, waist measurement, physical fitness	T=↓ weight, BMI, waist measure compared to C at post-test	Small sample, targets high prevalence group; endorses individual empowerment as change strategy

(continued)

Table 4.1 Interventions in obesity (continued)

Author (year)	Objective	Design	Intervention	Mode	Sample	Outcome measures	Results	Notes
Carels et al. (2007)	Evaluate MI with weight loss program on weight loss	RCT 2-matched group, comparison, pre-post design; T1 = MI + weight loss program; T2 = weight loss program only	T1 & T2 = weight loss program in 12 (1 hour) sessions; T1 included individual sessions of MI	Small group + individual	T1 = 28; 85% women; 93% white; 2/3 college degree & married; T2 = 24; 89% women, 92% white, 59% college, 70% married	Weight loss, diet improvement, physical activity	T1 = ↓ weight loss & ↑ physical activity over T1 group	Small sample limits, but detailed steps in maintaining integrity of MI is very useful for replication
Channon et al. (2007)	Evaluate MI on weight loss with Type 1 diabetic adolescents	RCT 2-group, pre-post 6, 12, & 24 months; design; T = MI; C = support visit	MI sessions over 12 months to motivate weight loss & dietary control	Individual	All white & averaged 15 y/o; T = 38, 47% female; C = 28; 50% female	Weight loss, depression, & anxiety	T = ↓ anxiety & depression, & weight with maintenance over 24 month study compared to C	Small sample, but evidences promise of MI with teens
Dreimane et al. (2007)	Evaluate a behavioral change weight loss program with children, teens & parents	RCT 2-group, comparison, pre-post test design	Weekly 90 minute sessions T1 = 8 week T2 = 12 week	Small group for teens and small group for parents	7–17 y/os: T1 = 180 T2 = 84	Weight, height, BMI, health status, emotional & self-esteem; family cohesion scales	T1 ↑ weight loss compared to T2; those with higher self-esteem lost more weight in both groups	Large sample but shows efficacy of cost-effective shorter term intervention

Hildebrandt (1998)	Evaluate a support group for post-bariatric surgery clients	Non-random, convenience retrospective 2-group design; T=attended support group; C=did not attend	Support group	Small open group	Sample of 69 bariatric patients	Weight loss since surgery	Attenders reported greater weight loss than non-attenders	Very limited due to lack of randomization, voluntary participation, and self-report retrospectively
Painot et al. (2001)	Evaluate nutrition & CBT intervention on weight loss	RCT comparison 2-group, pre-post test design. T1=nutrition + CBT; T2=CBT alone	Nutritional education and CBT on nutrition & diet in 12-week program		Sample all women & white, averaging 42 years of age; T1=25 T2=35	Daily food diaries, daily weight, Eating Disorders Inventory, Hospital Anxiety & Depression, & Beck Depression Inventory	T1 ↑ weight loss, & psychological measures compared to T2	Small & all white sample, but endorses combined approach

(continued)

Table 4.1 Interventions in obesity (continued)

Author (year)	Objective	Design	Intervention	Mode	Sample	Outcome measures	Results	Notes
Perri et al. (2001)	Evaluated 3 behavioral therapy (BT) interventions on maintaining weight loss among obese women	RCT 3 group, pre-post & follow-up at 6 & 12 month design; randomized after BT; T1 = BT; T2 = BT + relapse prevention (RPT); T3 = BT + problem solving therapy (PST)	All completed BT in 5-month, 20 session program on nutrition & goal setting, weight management; RPT on support & education; PST on coping skills, & problem solving strategies	Small group	All women (N = 80) aged 21–60 y/os; T1 = 15; T2 = 20; T3 = 23 (does not provide demographics of each group)	Weight, weight loss & weight loss maintenance	T3 ↑ weight loss & ↑ maintenance over both T1 and T2	Small sample size is limiting; interventions appropriate to social work & design is supportive
Resnicow et al. (2001)	Evaluate MI on eating patterns in culturally shaped intervention in 14 Black churches	RCT 3-group comparison, post 12 month design; T1 = cultural program + 1 phone call; T2 = cultural program + 4 phone calls using MI T3 = cultural program only	Cutlurally shaped program included video, & pastor discussions on health eating with spiritual themes	Small group + individual	Sample 73% female, aged on average 44 years; 54% married; no details of each group given	Dietary daily journal; log for intake of fruits & vegetables	T2 ↑greater changes in healthy eating patterns at follow-up than either T1 or T3	Small sample, but supports import of cultural salience in interventions; details of intervention provided clearly

Study	Purpose	Design	Intervention	Format	Sample	Measures	Outcomes	Comments
Smith-West et al. (2007)	Evaluate MI intervention on weight loss among overweight diabetics	RCT 2-group comparison, pre & multiple post measure design; T1=42 session weight loss program + MI; T2=health topics in 5 sessions	5 sessions of MI over 12 months	Small group	Sample N=217, average age 54, 1/3 African American, 2/3 employed; T1=109 T2=108	Weight, height, attendance in weight loss program, food & exercise diaries	T1 ↑ weight loss & maintenance at 6, 12 & 18 month follow up compared to T2	Further evidence of efficacy of MI; extensive details of interventions provided
Welch et al. (2008)	Evaluate a post-bariatric surgery support group	Non-random 2-group retrospective comparison, T=support group; C=regular post-op care alone	Support group on adherence to diet & behaviors & physical activity	Small group	Sample 89% women, 61% married, 81% white; T=200 C=100	Self-report food diaries & adherence to post Bariatric regimens	More in the T group maintained weight loss & adhered to regimen than in the control group	Limited by non-random, retrospective design and small sample; suggest that post-op long term intervention may be helpful in maintenance post-op
Yin et al. (2005)	Evaluate an interactional multi-component intervention with obese 4th graders	RCT 2-group pre-test/post-test design; T=66; C=52	Intervention conversational & interactional based on issues of each child & session	Small group	N=118; T=56% male, average age 9.4 years; C=54% male, average age 94 years	BMI, skin fold thickness, weight loss, dietary knowledge & attitude & behavior related to weight loss	T=↑ knowledge, & behaviors at post-test compared to C. No change in weight loss or weight for height index.	One of the very few studies evaluating interventions with obese children. Small sample is limiting; extensive details of interactional content provided

Notes: T = intervention/treatment group; T1 = 1st intervention group; T2 = 2nd intervention group; T3 = 3rd intervention group; C = control or comparison group; UC = usual care (e.g., physician visit, medication); BMI = Body Mass Index.

Glossary

Bariatric surgery—surgical intervention in body on the organs of the body that function in ingestion, or nutritional absorption.

BMI—basal metabolism index; a measure of the proportion of fat in the body.

Chronic illness—an illness characterized by the following: a serious, ongoing health condition that has a biological, anatomical, or physiologic basis and has lasted, or is expected to last, at least one year.

Co-morbid/co-morbidity(ies)—conditions or disease that are associated with a disease or disorder.

Gastroplasty—surgical interventions in the organs of the gastric system of the body (e.g., stomach, intestines).

Incidence—the rate of an occurrence of a disease or disorder per a number of persons (i.e., 100,000 or 1,000).

Morbid obesity—a diagnosis that the BMI (class III) is equal to or greater than 40.0, risk factors, and waist circumference are extreme and weight is greater than 200 percent, or 100 pounds, over ideal weight for height.

Morbidity—any departure, subjective or objective, from a state of physical or psychological well being, may be expressed as a proportion of persons per 100,000 persons with a particular diagnosis or condition.

Mortality—the number of deaths in a given year per 100,000 persons in a defined population; the measure of the occurrence of death in a defined population during a specified interval of time.

Obese—a condition indicating that BMI is 30 kg/height, and the extent of body fat places an individual at risk for several health problems.

Overweight—a lay term generally used interchangeably with the term obese.

Prevalence—the proportion of a population having a disease, diagnosis, or medical condition over a specific period of time (e.g., year) expressed in a percentage.

Risk factor—an established direct cause of, or contributor to, the morbidity or mortality of a particular diagnosis or medical condition.

Sequela(ae)—an after effect of a disease, injury, procedure, or treatment.

A Scenario of being Overweight and Obese and Questions for Reflection and Discussion

Tamika Southwell is a 34 year old, who is married and employed full-time as an administrative assistant, in a corporation that manages several retirement centers in the region. Her husband is a co-owner in a local car dealership. The couple has two children; one daughter aged four years, and a son, aged seven years. Ms. Southwell is pre-diabetic, and has pre-hypertension. Her physician has told her that both conditions are exacerbated by her weight, and that both conditions would likely resolve were she to lose that weight. She is 65 pounds over what she should be for her height. The physician has referred her to you with the goal of her losing and maintaining the loss of the weight. Mr. Southwell, who is not overweight, brags about his wife's good cooking, especially her lasagne and fried chicken. Tamika tells you that she has been overweight since childhood, that all the women in her family are overweight and a few are obese. She jokes that it is their "heritage" to like food. She further explains that she works fulltime, and prides herself on her cooking, pleasing her husband and children, and her church activities. She also says that she has tried several times to lose weight, beginning during her teen years, but no matter what has always gained the weight back, and is grateful that her friends no longer tease her about her weight like her friends in high school did. She has considered going to exercise classes within her neighborhood, but "can't fit it in." She tells of paying to join a weight-loss program in the community and not ever actually getting there. She admits that her doctor "kind of scared me" about the diabetes and blood pressure, but that her mother has both, and is obese as well, and seems okay. She becomes uncomfortable when you ask if her children are overweight at all.

1) What are the psychosocial stressors influencing Ms. Southwell and the challenge of losing weight at present?
2) a) What knowledge about weight and obesity and the physical risks of each would you share with her?
   b) What promising interventions for work with Tamika would you select, and what is your rationale for that choice or choices?
   c) Would you involve her husband and/or her children and/or her family members in your work with her?
3) How would your responses to each #1 and #2 of the above vary, or not, were Ms. Southwell a male African American of the same age, married with two children, and with the same degree of being overweight?
4) a) How would you respond differently to each #1 and #2 of the above, or not, were Tamika, instead of being an adult, 14 years of age?

    b) How would the age of the identified client revise the interventions you would select?

5) How would you respond to #1 and #2 of the above had the physician referred Ms. Southwell and her oldest child to you because the child is overweight, approaching obese status?

5   Pediatric Cancer

◆   Who is affected by pediatric cancer?
◆   What is childhood cancer and what types affect children
    and youth?
◆   What are the associated medical regimens and treatments?
◆   What psychosocial stressors are associated for families,
    children, and adolescents?
◆   What interventions are promising for social work
    implementation?
    •   Family- or parent-focused interventions
    •   Child- and adolescent-focused interventions
◆   Glossary
◆   Scenario

Introduction

The image of cancer in childhood and adolescence elicits strong
emotional responses even among those never having experienced the
disease in their family or friends. The image of a "terminal" illness
prompts anxieties and fear in general. However, the prospect of what is
perceived as a terminal illness in children and youth is almost more than
can be calmly understood. However, the mortality rates in pediatric
cancer over recent decades have improved greatly with consistent
increase, and more major investments in research, and in the development of medical and pharmaceutical interventions. The psychosocial
impact at diagnosis is historically the focus of pediatric cancer research.
Currently, because of increasing survival rates, the psychosocial sequelae
of surviving pediatric cancer prompt research into the survivor experience as it impacts child and youth survivors in psychological, emotional,
and developmental terms. As survivorship increases, pediatric cancer
survivors throughout their lives, and/or their families may seek care at
various times and for various issues after the event of diagnosis itself
during childhood. Accordingly, this chapter seeks to provide the best
practices for intervening during diagnostic and treatment phases, and
during survival years.

For practitioners to practice effectively with these clients and client systems, some background about the rates, types, and treatments for cancer in childhood and youth is necessary. Thus, this chapter first discusses the incidence and characteristics of the affected population, types of cancer commonly found in this population, related medical treatments, and the psychosocial stressors on the families and their offspring of a diagnosis of cancer during childhood and youth. Following this background, the details of the six studies on interventions identified in the systematic review that have promise of efficacy are discussed. The chapter concludes with a brief exploration of implications for practice and future research, a glossary of relevant terms, and a scenario on pediatric cancer and questions for reflection and discussion.

Who Is Affected by Cancer in Children

Rather than prevalence rates, incidence rates are used in pediatric cancer. An incidence rate is an estimate of the number of diagnoses per a population size (e.g., 100,000), rather than the proportion of a population having a disease or diagnosis as in prevalence rates. Incidence rates of a disease are often also reported separately by age groups, or gender, or racial and ethnic populations, and for specific types of a disease. The National Cancer Institute (NCI), for instance, reports the incidence rate, changes in that rate, and survival rates for all cancers, including pediatric cancer (2006b). In relation to this chapter, the Institute (2006a) reported that, in 2000, 10,400 children (15 years of age and less) in the U.S. had a diagnosis of cancer, of which approximately 15 percent would die of the disease. The NCI estimates the incidence rate for cancer among children 14 years of age and younger at one to two per 10,000 children in America (2006b). Though these numbers are clearly small, the disease is the leading cause of death due to disease among children, and is second only to accidents.

On a happier note, the overall survival rates for children have increased since the mid-1970s (28 percent) such that at present three-quarters to four-fifths will survive (NCI, 2006b; Patenaude & Kupst, 2005; Schwartz, 2003). Survival estimates are based on the criteria that no cancer is present for at least a five-year period after the initial diagnosis. The improvement in survival rates for pediatric cancer have come about from intense funding and research in various types of pediatric cancers, the ongoing development of treatments and pharmaceuticals for these cancers, and the establishment of cancer centers devoted to the research, treatment, and clinical trials on children and teens with cancer (e.g., St. Jude's) (NCI, 2006a; 2006b). Survival rates for some specific types of cancers in children and youth exceed the overall current estimated survival rate; examples of these are brain and nervous system cancers (74 percent), kidney cancer (i.e., Wilms tumor; 92 percent), and Hodgkin lymphoma (95 percent) (NCI, 2006b).

The NCI identifies white, non-Hispanic children as being the most likely among racial and ethnic groups to have some type of cancer (2006b). The incidence rates of childhood malignancies by age group begin in rates during infancy, which represent 10 percent of all pediatric cancers in those under 15 years of age. Incidence rates are the highest in the northeastern region of the country (Centers for Disease Control & Prevention, 2005b). According to the Centers for Disease Control & Prevention (2005b), during the period 1990 to 2004 the mortality rates for boys from cancer (33.1: 1 million) was significantly greater than among girls (26: 1 million) and for whites (30:1 million) and blacks (29.3: 1 million) compared to other racial populations. Mortality rates vary regionally as well; the mortality rate for pediatric cancer is higher in the western region of the U.S.

The incidence rates for cancer among adolescents (15 to 19 years of age) is estimated by the NCI as 202.2 per million, much greater than the rate among five to nine (110.2: 1 million) or ten to 14 year olds (117.3: 1 million) (2006b). In addition, variances by gender in adolescence are distinct. The overall incidence of cancer among teen boys, for instance, is reported by the NCI as 120 percent greater than among younger cohort males; thyroid cancer is more common among female than among male adolescents (2006a; 2006b).

What Is Pediatric Cancer?

Extensive research into the cause or causes of pediatric cancer indicates that it is likely that a mutated gene or genes are involved in most pediatric cancers, but not through an inherited or inheritable genetic mutation. Rather, the National Cancer Institute (2006a) in discussing changes (mutations) in genes that lead to pediatric cancer note that these changes occur early in life, in an *acquired* mutation. This type of mutation ensues when one cell in the normal process of cell development mutates and passes on that change to the cells that come from that original cell in cell division. The process of cell division and development occurs in the fetus, and continues throughout life. One illustration of the role of cell development in pediatric cancer might be seen by comparing the incidence rates of germ cell carcinoma, such as gonadal tumors, in adolescence (30.8: 1 million) with those of younger cohorts (less than 7: 1 million) (2006a). The role of *acquired* mutations is very different from what is known currently about genetic links with some cancers of adulthood (e.g., breast cancer). Similarly, while risk factors in lifestyle are major factors in cancer in adulthood (e.g., diet, smoking), no lifestyle risk factors for cancers in childhood and adolescence have been identified at present (NCI, 2006a; 2006b).

The kinds of cancers of childhood and adolescence tend to be different from the cancers of adulthood. The common pediatric cancers include, for example, leukemias, brain and nervous system tumors, lymphomas, bone cancers, and kidney cancers (NCI, 2006b), each of which are significantly less common in adulthood. The predominate types of cancers among adolescents are Hodgkin's disease and germ cell, particularly greater among teens aged 15 to 19 years than earlier in adolescence.

Among the 12 major types of childhood cancers, leukemias (blood cell cancers) and cancers of the brain and nervous system account for more than half of new cases; about one-third of all childhood cancers are leukemias (NCI, 2006b). The most common type of leukemia in children is acute lymphoblastic leukemia (ALL). The most common solid tumors are brain tumors. In order of prevalence, the types of pediatric cancers are:

- leukemias,
- brain and nervous system cancers,
- neuroblastoma,
- Wilms tumor,
- lymphoma.

In brief, leukemias are cancers of blood cells, and are the most common of all cancers in children (about one-third). Leukemias cause pain in bones and joints, generalized weakness, and fever, among other symptoms. Brain and nervous system (central nervous system; CNS) cancers—the second largest group of childhood cancers, comprising about one-fifth of childhood cancers—usually affect the cerebellum or the stem of the brain. Symptoms include headaches, vision problems, difficulty in walking, or in the use of the hands. Two other types of cancers comprise smaller proportions; these are neuroblastoma (7 percent) and Wilms tumor (5 percent). Neuroblastoma is a solid tumor, most often found in the abdomen, and typically occurring in infancy before the age of one. Wilms tumor, predominately occurring among two- to three-year-old children, is a tumor of one or both kidneys. Lymphomas are either Hodgkin's or non-Hodgkin's lymphomas that begin in lymphatic tissues, and spread to other areas, such as bone marrow (4 percent).

The NCI SEER reports (2006b) that the types of cancers most prevalent among adolescents differ from the types most prevalent among younger cohorts. That is, the most common cancer among teens is Hodgkin's (16 percent), followed by germ cell tumors (15.2 percent), and central nervous system tumors (10.0 percent).

Medical Treatment in Pediatric Oncology

The course of medical treatments for any type of cancer—combinations of chemotherapies, radiation, and/or surgery—are determined by the type, location, and stage of the cancer. Both chemotherapy and radiation therapy are delivered over a specified period and dose calibrated to the type and location(s) of the cancers. In general, chemotherapy has proven effective in most types of pediatric cancers, possibly due to the rapidity of growth in these cancers. Chemotherapy is the infusion of pharmaceuticals that literally kill the cancer cells. The infusions are delivered over the course of several days. As such, these chemicals cause predictable unpleasant, often seriously unpleasant, side effects. Among the side effects are nausea and vomiting, pain, and fatigue, each of which may be extreme. While medications can alleviate each of these side effects, recent literature suggests that these three side effects are actually linked (Davies, Whitsett, Bruce, & McCarthy, 2002; Whitsett, Gudmundsdottir, Davies, McCarthy, & Friedman, 2008). Further, Whitsett and colleagues (2008) report that the fatigue associated with chemotherapy is not resolved through sleep or rest, and is associated with feelings of isolation, worry, and/or depression in pediatric cancer patients.

Radiation therapy (RT), a painless and non-invasive treatment for pediatric cancer, may be used alone or as a co-therapy with surgery and/ or with chemotherapy and requires multiple doses over one to several weeks (Klosky et al., 2004). When used, this treatment requires practice sessions (i.e., no actual radiation occurs) to identify specific sites for radiation, and to create specific positioning devices for the patient. Multiple practice sessions may be necessary, each of which can last up to one and one-half hours, to make sure that, when radiation is implemented, the target site of the radiation is precise. Fewer complications from RT, including damage to healthy tissue, acute and/or chronic side effects, and the need to use sedation medications or anesthesia, are reduced when positioning is maintained (Zhu, Stovall, Buter, Ji, Gaber, & Samant, 2000). The use of sedation and anesthesia, because, in children especially, it is associated with medical risks for complications, is to be avoided in favor of behavioral interventions to maintain correct positioning of the child.

The settings of pediatric oncology services deserve some attention in this discussion as they differ from what is generally thought of as hospital-based care. The usual care provided in the 25 childhood cancer treatment centers in the nation are multidisciplinary and highly coordinated teams of pediatric oncologists, radiation specialists, oncology nurses and practitioners, psychologists, social workers, rehabilitation experts, pastoral counselors, and educators (Foreman, Willis, & Goodenough, 2005; Sahler et al., 2005). In contrast to usual care in general or regional hospitals, care in cancer specialty centers is ongoing and supportive, and seeks to provide involvement and support to the family and the child in each of the emotional, financial, and care realms. The transdisciplinary perspective of this care locates the child and her/his family at the center of care provided.

Psychosocial Stress in Parents, Families, Children, and Teens

The literature discussing stress and cancer during childhood describes stressors in the context of a continuum: disease, diagnosis, treatment, and survival. Intervening within the context of those phases is both appropriate and linked to efficacy (Kazak, 2005). The literature indicates that responses of the child, youth, and of their parents and families, during the initial diagnostic and treatment period appear to diminish over time for most.

Kazak and Baxt (2007) note that the reactions of families throughout the process arise from the intensity of the child's illness, the impact of the illness on pre-existing family relationships, responsibilities, and roles. Additionally, families' capacities for coping, adaptation, and adjustment fluctuate in relation to the point in the continuum of care in which the family finds itself. In illustration, a family's responses, and coping strategies during testing and diagnosis are most likely anxious, feeling overwhelmed and possibly depressed. As care and treatments evolve, the family adjusts while attending to the ongoing needs of all the members of the family. Kazak and Baxt (2007) report that a consistent portion, one-quarter to one-third, of the children and their families experience significant problems in family relationships, in individual member's difficulties, in psychological well-being, and/or in social contexts. The social contexts that may be or may become challenging to families and their child are schools, parents' employment, and dysfunctional social relationships outside the family. Varni, Katz, Colegrove, and Dolgin (1993) explore the challenges in social and school settings for children diagnosed with cancer. The obvious challenge arises from absences from school during diagnosis and initial treatments. Those authors emphasize the need for re-integration into school as soon as medically appropriate. However, re-adjustment to school is not a simple accomplishment, and one which can be challenged once again when, and if the child or teen is absent because of needed further treatments, and/or follow up care. In both the initial re-entry and any subsequent re-entries, social support and acceptance of school peers and of teachers are opportunities for the child to return to a normal lifestyle, and are essential to successful re-integration. As Varni and co-authors remind, the child's perception of being accepted and socially supported mitigate against their feeling isolated, the latter being associated with increased anxiety in the child. In sum, the psychosocial environment of the school, as is normative for non-cancer children and youth, is also central to the child or teen with cancer rejoining peers, and achieving goals both academically and developmentally.

Long-term effects can be psychosocial and/or physical sequelae of the cancer or its treatment. These latter, known as "late effects," can include difficulties in bio-psychosocial domains, and persist into and throughout adulthood (Friedman & Meadows, 2002). Kazak (2005), Patenaude and Kupst (2005), and Dolgin, Somer, Buchvald, and Zaizov (1999) describe the late effects of having cancer early in life. They posit that late effects are related to the further developmental milestones in the child or teen (e.g., school achievement, relationship building with peers, employment), and to the problems of parents and family members (e.g., disruptions in familial and marital relationships, anxieties, depression) (e.g., Kazak, 2005; Zebrack, Chesler, Orbuch, & Parry, 2002).

Parents, particularly mothers, are reported to experience ongoing or recurring anxieties and depression (Kazak & Baxt, 2007; Sahler et al., 2005). Anxieties of mothers are reported to be related to the demands of daily medical care for their child, fears of death, strains of the costs of the medical care, and possibly disrupted relationships within the family. The research of Zebrack, Chesler, et al. (2002) on the experience of mothers of survivors of pediatric cancer in a convenience sample used self-report questionnaires and individual interviews. Their content analysis of the transcribed interviews revealed three categories of worries: first, worries about the potentials of their child's relapse, second, worries about what they perceived as their child's worries, and third, worries about the meanings the mothers attached to their own and their child's experience of pediatric cancer. Implications for intervening with survivors and their mothers as well as other family members as noted by Zebrack and co-authors are psychosocial interventions that target worries about treatment during the treatment phase and ongoing small group and individual interventions on late effects in developmental, psychological, and psychosocial realms. The authors also recommend that all interventions with mothers include fathers and emphasize the research findings indicating the likelihood that pediatric cancer survivors do well in these domains.

Kazak and Baxt (2007) and Kazak et al. (1997), utilizing a PTSD conceptual framework, describe the reactions of the family to their child or teen's diagnosis as a response to a traumatic event. In this framework, the diagnosis of cancer is a life-threatening occurrence, a central concept of PTSD theory. Of course, cancer treatments can be not only painful, but in themselves can also threaten life. Kazak and Baxt describe the symptoms of PTSD as an intensity of fear and helplessness around the trauma event, with intrusive thoughts (re-experiencing), denial or numbing, and arousal (e.g., sleep problems). They link these symptoms of PTSD to the psychological sequelae of childhood cancer. Kazak and Baxt further suggest that the majority of diagnosed children and teens, and their families experience these types of symptoms at some point after the initial diagnostic, and treatment phases. One example reporting similar findings is that of Weiner et al. (2006). This research involved a small, retrospective study of 34 post-childhood cancer survivors (up to 17 years after the conclusion of treatment for sarcoma). Weiner et al. report that

77 percent of the participants scored in the clinically significant range of the Brief Symptom Inventory with stress indicators including intrusive thoughts, difficulty in adjusting to school and/or work, and worries about current health. In a very early cross-sectional study, Koocher and O'Malley (1981) found that about one-quarter of the survivors had impairments in some social functioning realms. Conversely, Zebrack, Zeltzer, Whitton, Mertens, Odom, and Berkow (2002), and others (Patenaude & Kupst, 2005) report that one-half to a majority of survivors of pediatric cancer do fairly well and are very similar in indicators of self-esteem, depression, and anxiety to the norms in their non-cancer age cohorts.

Extending the study of psychosocial stressors to the role of parents in the context of in-hospital and home-based treatment of their children diagnosed with cancer, Clark and Fletcher (2003) argue that the context of the care is essential in understanding the stressors on the family. Clark and Fletcher studied the influences and issues of the context of care with a convenience, snowball sample of voluntary parents whose child had cancer in lengthy qualitative interviews. Thematic content analysis revealed that the quality of parents' communication with professionals in the care of their child is the central issue of concern, in what the authors describe as a paradox of parents having and not having responsibility and authority in their child's care. This duality is exacerbated, according to Clark and Fletcher, by the expertise of medical and nursing personnel about the child's cancer, and the expectation of professionals that their relationships with parents is by nature of their professional expertise unequal (experts versus parents). The researchers link the imbalance of this relationship to the stress of parents. The authors suggest professional behaviors, such as listening to the patient and to their family, were related to enhancing health promoting behaviors of the child and the family.

Quin's 2004 study of the psychosocial outcomes of childhood cancer found that the majority of parents, survivors of pediatric cancer, and their siblings made positive adjustment after the completion of cancer treatment. Her study with 74 mothers, 46 fathers, 38 siblings and 42 survivors of childhood cancer in Ireland, used multiple specific and validated instruments for parents, for the children, and for siblings, and qualitative interviews. Quin relates findings identifying instrumental and emotional social support, turning to religious faith and acceptance as primary coping strategies. The support of family and extended family members was pivotal to coping during the diagnosis and treatment phases. In fact, several family members reported that the point at the conclusion of treatment was the most acutely stressful as they felt isolated and alone. In addition to participants evidencing adjustment, a few parents and children experienced ongoing problems. Of particular import for practitioners, this subgroup largely involved the cancer diagnosis occurring near or during adolescence. This finding has import for practitioners' identification of those families needing psychosocial long-term follow-up work.

Zebrack and colleagues (2002; 2004) have examined the psychological health of adult survivors of pediatric cancer in a national and ongoing study of survivors. The earlier study (Zebrack, Zeltzer, et al., 2002) involved adult survivors of pediatric leukemia, Hodgkin's disease, and non-Hodgkin's lymphoma and their siblings. A large sample (2,565) of the survivors and their siblings completed a questionnaire based on the Brief Symptom Inventory. Analysis revealed that the majority of those in the study did not indicate symptoms of depression. The survivors, in comparison to their siblings, more often indicated symptoms of depression, and women in both groups indicated significantly more often that they had symptoms of depression than men. The 2004 research sampled survivors (1,102) of pediatric brain cancer and their siblings (2,817). This latter study's findings were similar to the earlier work in that only a minority of survivors (11 percent) and even fewer among their siblings (5 percent) reported clinically significant symptoms of psychological problems. However, among survivors increased levels of depression, somatic complaints, and anxiety were significantly related to being female, unmarried, less educated, and unemployed. In conclusion, Zebrack and co-authors note that while survival of pediatric cancer does not appear to be related by itself to poorer mental health, the psychosocial and social functioning associated with cancer survivorship does. The latter supports the need for practitioners to be knowledgeable of the psychosocial issues related to being a survivor and being alert to indirect linkages to being a survivor of pediatric cancer.

In sum, both the articles by Quin (2004) and by Clark and Fletcher (2003) are invaluable for practitioners who wish to understand fully the psychosocial context and influences within which the families and children of pediatric oncology experience the disease, treatment, and post-treatment. Of significance for social workers, Patenaude and Kupst (2005) address the research reporting that survivors demonstrate little or no evidence of problems in anxiety, depression, or self-esteem in comparison to age-cohort population norms. Resultantly Patenaude and Kupst (2005) encourage practitioners to work with survivors and their families who are having difficulties from a strengths and competency perspective. In a similar vein, Casillas, Zebrack, and Zeltzer (2006), based on their study of Latino survivors of childhood cancer, encourage professionals to recognize and incorporate cultural strengths, and resilience factors, and the cultural salience of including not only the immediate family, but also extended family members in work with Latino survivors.

Zebrack and Chesler (2002) suggest that the experience of surviving cancer may enhance resilience, a resilience that is moderated, however, by concerns about whether the cancer will recur. Research to date suggests, however, that the episodic experience of stressors along the continuum of diagnosis, treatment, and survivorship can be severe in the short-term, and can have inter-linked associations and consequences in adult survivorship. In each instance, social worker skills in effective interventions are prerequisites for beneficial outcomes.

Taken together, the extensive literature and research suggests that the psychosocial stressors associated with pediatric cancer occur in varying degrees along the continuum of diagnosis, treatment, and survivorship, and in relation to the developmental stage of the survivor (e.g., Casillas et al., 2006). In light of the rising likelihood that teens and children will survive their cancer, the challenge now is to know what intervention works, and for whom, and then at what point in time that intervention is appropriate.

Promising Interventions with Children, Teens, Parents, and Families

Though research in the area of pediatric oncology has a substantial history, going back into the early 1970s, a substantial focus on psycho-social interventions is of comparatively recent origin. This latter is largely due to the improvements in the survivorship of children and youth with cancer discussed earlier in this chapter. Thus, it is not surprising that the empirical basis for efficacious psychosocial interventions with this popu-lation is comparatively small. Nonetheless, studies of psychosocial inter-ventions evidencing promise were located in this systematic review; these studies are discussed below.

Kazak et al. (2005) revised and evaluated their original SCCIP interven-tion (2004) in a randomized wait-list controlled study with the parents and caregivers of newly diagnosed children. Very similar to the original intervention, SCCIP-ND consisted of a four-session (one day) interven-tion combining cognitive behavioral and family therapy in a program, *Surviving Cancer Competently Intervention Program-Newly Diagnosed* (SCCIP-ND), plus individual family sessions. Thirty-eight parents/caregiv-ers were randomized to the treatment (nine families) or control group (ten families), the latter receiving only usual care. The SCCIP-ND version sought to assist families whose adolescent had cancer to reduce the impact of the diagnosis and treatment experiences through cognitive behavioral interventions. The intervention targeted the stress symptoms of PTSD, such as intrusive thoughts, avoidance, and arousal; measurements included acute stress disorder, impact of events, and state-trait anxiety validated scales, and staff monitoring forms. SCCIP-ND combines cogni-tive behavioral and family therapy as the earlier study did, in four sessions. Components of the four sessions were joining with the family, stressing the importance of the relationship between parents'/caregivers' effective coping and their child's progress, normalizing family experiences, and focusing on the strengths of the family. Mini-scenarios from video tapes of live multi-family group sessions of pediatric cancer parents and caregivers were incorporated in the individual family sessions to prompt attention to the experiences of other families, and the normative issues that arise. Due to the small sample size, findings are depicted graphically showing that the treatment group's state anxiety and post-traumatic stress symptoms scores decreased between baseline and post-interventions points while those of the control group did not.

Sahler and colleagues (2005) studied the effect on mothers of newly diagnosed children of a usual psychosocial care plus problem solving skills training (PSST; T1) compared with usual psychosocial care alone (T2) in seven cancer center sites across the country. Participants were randomly assigned to the combined (n = 217) or the usual care (n = 213) intervention groups. The average age of the participating mothers was 35 and 32 years respectively in T1 and T2; overall two-thirds were married, about one-half were white, and less than one-tenth were African American. The outcomes were assessed at baseline before randomization, at post-intervention and at three-month follow up points. Measurements included the following validated scales: NEO-FFI a multi-dimensional scale on personality traits of Extraversion, Agreeableness, and Conscientiousness; the revised Social Problem-Solving Inventory that summates in a functional and a dysfunctional problem solving skill score; the Profile of Mood States; the Impact of Event Scale that measures perceived posttraumatic stress negative affect; and the Beck Depression Inventory (BDI). PSST was a cognitive behavioral intervention conceptually based on problem solving therapy.

The study was framed by the concept that mothers of children with cancer are at increased risk of acute stress and that this stress is related to the daily responsibility of overseeing their child's medical care either in the hospital or in home-based after care including chemotherapy and medications. As described by Sahler and colleagues usual psychosocial care was a multi-disciplinary (e.g., medical, nursing, social work, psychology, psychiatry) approach designed to address the psychosocial, emotional, and care concerns of parents, siblings, and other affected members of the child's family system. The PSST intervention was an eight session (one hour each) intervention with individual mothers focusing on coping skills for the issues identified by each mother in each session; the intervention followed guidelines developed previously (Sahler et al., 2002; Varni et al., 1999).

Findings demonstrated that the mothers in the PSST intervention had significantly improved problem solving skills, and reduced negative feelings. Sahler and colleagues suggest that the promise of the PSST approach combined with usual care may deter the longer-term effects of the stress on the mother of a child diagnosed with cancer. The authors provide detailed tables and discussion of the intervention sessions that is of particular utility to practitioners wishing to plan and implement the combined intervention.

A study evaluated an intervention to reduce distress in the child during their radiation therapy (RT) for cancer (Klosky et al., 2004) in a sample of 79 children who were randomly assigned to an intervention group (n = 41) or a modified control group (n = 38). The children in the full sample were on average four years of age (4.2 years), largely non-Hispanic white (73.4 percent), and one-fifth African American (21.5 percent), over one-half of whom were boys (53.2 percent). The intervention group received a combined CBT package including an interactive-educational component. The latter, a seven-minute video capturing modeling during an RT treatment, features *Barney* and a young child actor that reinforces the optimal behaviors of children during radiation therapy through narrated stories. The video emphasizes the treatment, the machines used in the treatment, and the importance of staying very still during the procedure. An actual *Barney* (a 13-inch plush character doll) accompanies the child throughout the RT procedure. The child can animate the *Barney* by pushing buttons on the character doll's hands. Children in the modified comparison group received a similar intervention with a non-interactive character *Barney*, an unrelated cartoon-video of the child's choice, and stories unrelated to radiation therapy delivered via audiotape during the procedure. The outcome measures of the children in the pre-test/post-test design were the use of sedation, behavioral distress as indicated on the Observation Scale of Behavioral Distress (OSBD) scale, and heart rate. The OSBD is a 12-item scale reflecting the experience of the child at the time, such as saying that they were scared, telling the staff to stop, and crying; attending clinical staff that were trained in the use of the scale indicated such occurrences on the scale. Heart rate was recorded with a pulse finger oxisensor. Analysis comparing the two groups showed that the heart rate of children in the interactive group was significantly decreased, but that the use of sedation and observations of distress did not differ between the groups. As the authors indicate, the interactive intervention shows promise for effectively reducing the stress children experience during radiation therapy, but that studies are indicated that include pure control groups.

Building upon their earlier study on child outcomes (2004), Klosky, Garces-Webb, Buscemi, Schum, Tyc, & Merchant (2007) evaluated the effect of an interactive educational program on parent outcomes measuring anxiety and stress in relation to the radiation therapy procedures on their children in a pediatric cancer center. The study was conceptualized on the basis that parental distress and child distress during procedures such as RT are re-iterative with each affecting the other's levels of distress. The RCT two-group comparison design with 79 families were randomly assigned to either the interactive educational intervention (T1 = 41) or to a modified comparison (T2 = 39) group. The details of the *Barney* intervention package are supplied in the discussion of Klosky's 2004 study. In the 2007 study, all parents completed a standardized and validated state and trait anxiety scales (measuring how the parent felt and how they observed the child feeling during the treatment procedures) before randomization, and after the completion of all radiation treatments. The scores of the T1 intervention group were significantly improved in comparison to those of the T2 group. The discussion of the interventions in this study are particularly useful in developing and replicating the intervention in an area of central import for the psychosocial well being of the child and family in pediatric oncology, and ideally it is hoped in replicating the evaluation of the intervention. (See Table 5.1 for summarizations of the details of the promising interventions discussed in this chapter.)

An early RCT comparative two group, pre-post study evaluated social problem solving skills training among child survivors of cancer compared to a traditional intervention (Varni et al., 1993). Children, aged five to 13 years, previously diagnosed with cancer were randomly assigned to either a Social Skills Training (T1 = 33) or a School Re-integration Program (T2 = 31). The T1 and T2 groups were comparable in racial identification (51 percent and 45 percent non-Hispanic white, respectively) and about one-third of each group were African American, but varied in gender distribution (70 percent and 48 percent male, respectively). Overall, diagnostically about one-half of the children diagnosed with and treated for cancer had a diagnosis of acute lymphocytic leukemia.

The Social Skills Training intervention had three segments. These were: first, preventive education and support in the hospital concerning the importance and elements of transition back to school once discharged from the hospital including individual and family counseling; and second, presentations in the school with the child's peers, teachers, and school personnel including the children themselves; and third, routinely regular follow-up sessions over time with all participants. The researchers argued in their initial conceptual article that this highly structured approach is supported by research evidence on other illnesses post-diagnosis and treatment, and in such settings as schools (Katz & Varni, 1993). The T1 children had significantly increased perceived social support from peers and from teachers, and significantly decreased behavioral problems compared to T2 children at follow-up as indicated by their scores on the Internalizing and the Externalizing subscales of the Child Behavior Checklist (CBCL). Overall, this small study is supportive of school-based interventions and social skills training as a specific intervention with children post-diagnosis of cancer.

Kazak and colleagues pilot tested (1999), and then implemented, and evaluated (2004) an intervention in a RCT wait-list control trial with adolescent survivors of pediatric cancer survivors and their parents. Participants in the 2004 study were recruited from an oncology registry of adolescent patients who had completed treatment from one to ten years

Table 5.1 Interventions in pediatric cancer

Author (year)	Objective	Design	Intervention	Mode	Sample	Outcome measures	Results	Notes
Kazak et al. (2004)	Evaluate a stress reduction intervention with adolescent survivors, parents, & siblings	RCT 2-group waitlist control, pre-post design: stratified by age of teen (11–14 & 15–18); T1 = 76 (teens); C = 74 (teens)	One day 4-session on SCCIP; CBT & family systems therapy to reduce PTSD symptoms	Small group	N = 85% white; 1–10 years post completion of cancer treatment; 25% had leukemia; averaged 7.8 y/o at diagnosis	Impact of Events, PTSD-RI; State-Trait Anxiety, Children's Manifest Anxiety scales	T = fathers ↓ intrusive thoughts, mothers & teens ↓ arousal subscales compared to C at post-test	Extensive details of design & intervention
Kazak et al. (2005)	Evaluate an intervention to reduce stress in parents of children newly diagnosed with cancer (SCCIP-ND)	RCT 2-group, pre-post test design; T = SCCIP-ND; C = UC	SCCIP-ND is one day session of CBT + family therapy with video vignettes of MFG group sessions	Individual family	T = 9 families; C = 10 families; total of 38 parents/caregivers; diagnosed child's median age = 5 years (n = 19); 8 of 19 leukemia/lymphoma	Post trauma stress & anxiety, life events, & anxiety scales	T = ↓ PTSD & anxiety measures at post-test compared to C	Small sample, graphic analyses; one of the rare studies on the diagnosis phase of pediatric cancer
Klosky et al. (2004)	Evaluate child's stress during radiation	RCT 2-group comparison; T1 = interactive *Barney*; T2 = modified version with cartoon video of choice + non-interactive *Barney* doll	CBT + interactive video *Barney* showing role modeling just prior & during radiation + plush doll *Barney*	Individual child + parent	Child's average age = 4.2 years, 73% white, 21% African American, 53% male, 67% CNS cancer; T = 41; T2 = 38	Use of sedation, stress indicators (OSBD), pulse oximeter (heart rate)	T1 ↓ heart rate; no differences in sedation or OSBD	Limited by lack of control; creative intervention that needs controlled design further study

Study	Purpose	Design	Intervention	Modality	Sample	Measures	Results	Comments
Klosky et al. (2007)	Evaluate intervention to reduce parent stress during child's radiation therapy	RCT 2-group comparison, pre-post design; T1 = interactive *Barney*; T2 = modified version with cartoon video of choice + non-interactive *Barney* doll	CBT + interactive video *Barney* showing role modeling just prior & during radiation + plush *Barney* doll	Individual parent + child	79 families; T1 = 41; T2 = 39; children 47% female; 67% CNS cancer	Parental anxiety and stress with State Trait Anxiety Inventory (STAI)	↓ STAI scores in T1 compared to T2	Small sample; but one of rare studies during treatment phase of pediatric cancer; full details of intervention
Sahler et al. (2005)	Evaluate problem skills training (PSST) on mothers of children newly diagnosed in 7 cancer centers	RCT 2-group comparison, pre-post & post 3 months design; T1 = PSST; T2 = usual psychosocial care	PSST is a cognitive behavioral intervention + problem solving skills; 8 (1 hour) sessions	Individual	Sample: 2/3 married, 50% white; ~10% African American; T1 = 217; averaged 35 years old T2 = 213; averaged 32 years	Personality trait scale (NEO-FFI); social problem skill solving (SPSI); depression (BDI) scales	T1 = ↓ depression & negative emotions; ↑ problem solving skills compared to T2	Benefited by large, nationwide sample; a rarely studied phase of pediatric cancer; use of validated measures

(continued)

Table 5.1 Interventions in pediatric cancer (continued)

Author (year)	Objective	Design	Intervention	Mode	Sample	Outcome measures	Results	Notes
Varni et al. (1993)	Evaluate a social skills training program on children's re-integration into school after cancer treatment	RCT 2-group comparison, pre-post 6 & 9 month design; T1 = Social skills training (SST); T2 = School reintegration program	SST uses individual & family counseling, & coordinates with school during hospital stay trains in the school with child's peers, staff, & follows in regular sessions over time	Small group + individual and family counseling sessions	Sample age 5–13 years; ½ treated for acute lymphocitic leukemia; T1 = 33; 51% white; 70% male; T2 = 31; 45% white; 48% male	Multiple child measures (CDI, STAIC, SPPC, SSSC) on self-esteem, stress, & depression; parental CBCL	T1 = significantly ↑ perceptions of social support & ↓ behavior problems (CBCL) compared to T2 at all post-test points	Use of multiple validated measures, though small sample

Notes: T = intervention/treatment group; T1 = 1st intervention group; T2 = 2nd intervention group; T3 = 3rd intervention group; C = control or comparison group; UC = usual care (e.g., physician visit, medication); MFG = multi-family group; CBCL = Child Behavior Checklist.

earlier, had not relapsed, spoke English, and were geographically close enough to attend the session. A total of 142 mothers (T1 = 72, T2 = 70), 102 fathers (T = 157, T2 = 45), and 149 adolescent survivors (T1 = 50, T2 = 74) participated. One-half of the teens in the total sample were female, and 85 percent were non-Hispanic whites. The validated self-report measurement instruments were the Impact of Events Scale capturing PTSD constructs of intrusive thoughts, avoidance, and hyper-arousal; the PTSD-RI scale; the State-Trait Anxiety Inventory, a 40-item scale that captures current and dispositional anxiety; and the Revised Children's Manifest Anxiety Scale. Findings included that fathers in the intervention group had significantly improved symptoms of intrusion compared with the wait-list control group at post-test. Similarly, in comparison to the wait-list control group, survivors in the intervention group had significantly improved symptoms of arousal. The findings imply support for the intervention's efficacy in reducing symptoms of PTSD, and for family-centered interventions with teen survivors of cancer.

Implications for Practice and Future Research

The interventions with evidence of efficacy located in the systematic review of this text suggest that there are two categories of interventions worthy of replication. First, interventions with promise of efficacy and appropriate for social work practice were identified for implementation early in the continuum of pediatric cancer to ameliorate the stressors involved during the diagnostic and the treatment phases. Second, there is growing evidence for interventions that address the challenges of survivorship for school integration, and for reducing the results of the trauma of being diagnosed with cancer during childhood with several age groups of survivors. Some of these evaluative studies included diversity in their samples. However, greater diversity with attention given to the full cultural, familial, and psychosocial context of pediatric cancer children and adolescents, and of pediatric cancer survivors is warranted. The latter is particularly important given the statistics that project ongoing increasing numbers of survivors in general, and of long-term survivors. The possible psychosocial issues of adults, who when in childhood or adolescence were diagnosed with cancer, and survived the rigors of the disease and the extensive treatments involved, is not as yet the focus of intervention evaluative research, but needs to be.

On the positive side, the rigor and attention to detail in methodology, and in implementation, and refinement of the interventions discussed in this chapter help ensure that practitioners not only implement these interventions, but as they implement to evaluate the interventions for further promise of efficacy. Notably, the studies located and discussed in this chapter provide details of both to make it more likely that these next steps in evidence-based practice are more easily accomplished.

Glossary

Incidence—the rate of an occurrence of a disease or disorder per a specific number of persons (i.e., 100,000 or 1,000).

Leukemia—cancer of blood cells, or of blood cell production; is the most common among pediatric cancers.

Lymphoma—non-Hodgkin or Hodgkin lymphomas (Hodgkin or Hodgkin's disease) is a cancer originating in the lymphatic tissues/lymph gland(s).

Neuroblastoma—the most common solid tumor besides brain tumors in pediatric cancer; most often occurs within the first year of life.

Prevalence—the proportion of a population having a disease, diagnosis, or medical condition over a specific period (e.g., year) expressed as a percentage.

Risk factor—an established direct cause of, or contributor to, the morbidity or mortality of a particular diagnosis or medical condition.

Sarcoma(s)—a malignant tumor growing from connective tissues, such as cartilage, fat, muscle, or bone.

Sequela (ae)—an after effect of a disease, injury, procedure, or treatment.

Survival rates—in relation to cancer, this rate refers to the percentage of patients who live *at least* five years after their cancer is diagnosed.

Wilms tumor—a cancer of one or both kidneys.

A Scenario in Pediatric Cancer and Questions for Reflection and Discussion

Jamie is an eight-year-old boy who was diagnosed with leukemia one year ago, and treated in an urban pediatric cancer center approximately 120 miles from his home. He and his mother, 31-year-old Martina, stayed at the center for all of his treatment, which lasted just over five months in total. During that treatment, Jamie was on a home-visit once for about two weeks, just prior to his last chemotherapy series. Jamie was discharged from the center with a good prognosis three months ago. Jamie's family includes a younger sister (aged three years), and his parents, Martina and Pat (aged 32 years); his maternal grandmother is also living with the family as she did during Jamie's hospitalization. Pat is employed in a local manufacturing company as a shift manager (3–11 p.m.). They live in a small town, in a largely rural area of the state.

Prior to being diagnosed Jamie was in the last semester of the second grade of a consolidated school (kindergarten through high school). Some activities at the cancer center were related to schoolwork for the children; when he felt good, he participated in these. Martina recently called the cancer center to speak with you, a social worker at the center, with whom the family established a relationship. Martina wanted to talk about Jamie's returning to school in his community. The school was encouraging her to let him come back to the same second grade teacher he had when he left for his cancer treatment. Jamie is scheduled to return to the center in three months for a status checkup; these appointments will routinely occur every six months afterward, unless during an appointment it is found that the cancer has returned.

1) a) What are the psychosocial stressors with which Jamie and his family are currently dealing?
   b) What psychosocial issues around his re-entry to school at this time would you explain to Martina?
   c) What are the challenges related to his leukemia to accomplishing the tasks of Jamie's current developmental stage?
   d) How would you include, or not include information from research around Jamie's re-entry to school and surviving childhood leukemia?

2) Since the family lives 120 miles away, how would you develop a plan to assist them with Martina over the phone?

3) a) What interventions with promise of effectiveness would you use in working with Martina and her family concerning the question of Jamie's return to school?
   b) In what ways would you include Jamie's school in the process?

4)   a)   How might your responses to #1, #2, and #3 above differ were Jamie to be 18 years old and had continued to be cancer free since the time identified in the scenario, and planning on entering college?

     b)   How might your responses to #1, #2, and #3 above differ were Jamie a 25-year-old female, who also had remained cancer free?

     c)   In what ways would you alter your responses to #4a and 4b were the survivor of pediatric cancer Hispanic or African American?

Afterword

The text examined five diseases or conditions each of which have major life challenging and/or life threatening characteristics for populations that are expanding, and expected to continue to expand in the next decade. A total of 68 interventions with some promise of effectiveness in practice were located through extensive systematic searches of the major databases. An explication of each intervention was detailed, along with their implications for social work practice and research.

The goal of the text was to take a step toward providing practitioners with the best practices for social work in health concerning the major diseases that affect children, teens, families, and adults. Being a practitioner with the requisite skills and knowledge to intervene with these populations is both an ethical obligation to our clients, but also a responsibility to contribute to the advance of our profession.

The interventions discussed herein are particularly crucial to credible practice in health care for three reasons. One reason is that the world of health care is evermore demanding that we are credible practitioners among the professionals practicing in the transdisciplinary environment of health care. The second reason is quite practical. That is, managed care and third party payers demand that we demonstrate that what we "do" with clients has some evidence of effectiveness and that we can demonstrate that effectiveness with clients. Because of the latter, the text includes the methodology and designs, and their limitations, of the evaluative studies of each of the interventions discussed. It is the author's hope that the inclusion of methodological details can be used by practitioners to replicate not only the intervention, but to evaluate the intervention in their own practice.

To be an evidence-based practitioner, one must be able to analyze critically how well an intervention purposed to be efficacious fits our particular clients. In terms of the disease and conditions presented in this text, that requires a matching of the demographic characteristics, and settings in which the study occurred. Thus, these details of the interventions in this text include those details, when they were provided by the researchers. This issue further prompts that social workers in health care practice in the twenty-first century attend to the necessity of further research evaluating interventions with clients of diverse backgrounds and growing disease prevalence rates. The prevalence and incidence rates for some of the illnesses covered in the text speak directly to the need for further evidentiary research on interventions centering on diverse health care clients. Take this not as a daunting task! Rather, it is an opportunity for social workers to do what we have always done best—develop and evaluate interventions and approaches with the most vulnerable clients and client groups.

Appendix: Steps and Process of the Systematic Reviews

This text is based on systematic reviews of each of the identified health conditions, and diseases. The systematic reviews for each were conducted through the following processes. Details for each chapter follow this overview of the review processes.

Electronic searches were conducted with the following: PubMED, CINAHL (Cumulative Index to Nursing & Allied Health), PsychINFO, Social Work Abstracts, and the Cochrane Collaboration databases. Search terms were: (random OR control OR compar*) AND (interven* OR treatment) AND (psychosocial OR behavioral OR psychological OR coping). The "*" following "compare" allows the search to include forms of that word, such as, in this case, compare, compared, comparison. The search upon which each chapter in this text is based also included the following as relevant to the topic of each chapter: each illness or condition of interest, and population parameters as relevant (e.g., childhood, adolescence). All searches were limited to sources published in English and with human participants; no limit on years of the search was imposed in the first search. That first search occurred in May 2007; the exact same searches for each illness or condition were repeated for the interim period of 2007 through January 2009 in February of 2009.

Abstracts extracted through the search processes were examined, and the full article extracted if the abstract suggested that the study was eligible for inclusion among promising interventions of this text. Excluded were case studies, single group designs, studies with insufficient information for replication of the intervention, and reports of studies on the effect of medical outcomes only (e.g., drugs, chemotherapy). Each full article extracted as potentially eligible was then scrutinized for the following inclusion criteria: first, some level of effectiveness of the intervention, second, the intervention was appropriate for implementation by professional social workers; third, the study had at least one psychosocial, emotional, or psychological outcome, fourth, it included details of sample characteristics, settings, and design. The specific outcomes of the searches for each chapter are detailed below.

Asthma in Childhood and Adolescence

The search for interventions with some efficacy for children and teens with asthma included the terms asthma* and (child* OR adolescen* OR teen*). The database search located 234 studies potentially eligible; these abstracts were reviewed, and 72 possible studies were identified for possible inclusion in the review. The full articles of these studies were retrieved and scrutinized, resulting in the 22 studies meeting all the inclusion criteria. These interventions are discussed in Chapter 1 in detail and summarized in Table 1.1 and Table 1.2.

Diabetes

The search for promising interventions included the term diabet*; no restrictions on population characteristics were imposed. The database search for diabetes located 100 potentially eligible studies. These abstracts were reviewed, with identification of 55 possible studies for inclusion. The full articles of these studies were retrieved and scrutinized, resulting in the 20 studies meeting all the inclusion criteria. These interventions are discussed in Chapter 2 in detail and summarized in Table 2.1 and Table 2.2.

Hypertension

The search for promising interventions included the terms (hypertens* OR blood pressure OR high blood pressure OR elevated blood pressure); no restrictions on population characteristics were imposed. The database search located 69 potentially eligible studies. These abstracts were reviewed, with identification of 19 possible studies for inclusion. The full articles of these were retrieved and scrutinized, resulting in the eight studies meeting all the inclusion criteria. These interventions are discussed in Chapter 3 in detail and summarized in Table 3.1.

Obesity

The search for promising interventions included the terms (obes* OR overweight OR weight loss OR weight loss management); no restrictions on population characteristics were imposed. The database search for obesity located 38 potentially eligible studies. These abstracts were reviewed, with identification of possible studies for inclusion. The full articles of these were retrieved and scrutinized resulting in 12 studies meeting all the inclusion criteria. These interventions are discussed in Chapter 4 in detail and summarized in Table 4.1.

Pediatric Cancer

The search for promising interventions included the terms cancer AND (pediatric OR child* OR adolescent*) AND (family OR parents). The database search for pediatric cancer detected 62 potentially eligible studies. These abstracts were reviewed, with identification of 19 possible studies for inclusion. The full articles of these were retrieved and scrutinized, resulting in six studies meeting all the inclusion criteria. These interventions are discussed in Chapter 5 in detail and summarized in Table 5.1.

References

Adolfsson, E., Walker-Engstrom, M-L., Smide, B., & Wikblad, K. (2007). Patient education in type 2 diabetes—a randomized controlled 1-year follow-up study. *Diabetes Research and Clinical Practice, 76*, 341–350.

Agurs-Collins, C., Kumanyika, S., Have, T., & Adams-Campbell, L. (1997). A randomized controlled trial of weight loss and exercise for diabetic management in older African American women. *Diabetes Care, 20*(10), 1503–1511.

Akinbami, L. (2006). *The state of childhood asthma, United States, 1980–2005. Advance data from vital and health statistics,* No. 381. Hyattsville, MD: National Center for Health Statistics.

Akinbami, L., & Schoendorf, K. (2002). Trends in childhood asthma: Prevalence, health care utilization, and mortality. *Pediatrics, 110*(2), 315–322.

American Diabetes Association. (2005). *Facts and statistics.* Retrieved November 15, 2008 from http://www.diabetes.org/diabetes-statistics/prevalence.jsp.

American Lung Association, Epidemiology and Statistics Unit, Research and Program Services. (September 2007). Trends in asthma morbidity and mortality: Asthma & Children Fact Sheet. Retrieved November 11, 2008 from www.lungusa.org.

Anderson, B., Loughlin, C., Goldberg, E., & Laffel, L. (2001). Comprehensive, family-focused outpatient care for very young children living with chronic disease: Lessons from a program in pediatric diabetes. *Children's Services: Social Policy, Research, and Practice, 4*(4), 235–250.

Anderson, R., Funnell, M., Butler, P., Arnold, M., Fitzgerald, J., & Feste, C. (1993). Patient empowerment: Results of a randomized controlled trial. *Diabetes Care, 18*(7), 943–949.

Appel, L., Champagne, C., Harsha, D., Cooper, L., Obarzanek, E., Elmer, P. et al. (2003). Effects of comprehensive lifestyle modification on blood pressure control: Main results of the PREMIER clinical trial. *Journal of the American Medical Association, 289*(16), 2083–2093.

Aranda, M., & Knight, B. (1997). The influence of ethnicity and culture on the caregiver stress and coping process: A sociocultural review and analysis. *The Gerontologist, 17*(3), 342–354.

Askins, M., Sahler, J., Sheran, S., Fairclough, D., Butler, R., Katz, E. et al. (2008). Report from a multi-institutional randomized clinical trial examining computer-assisted problem-solving skills training for English-and Spanish-speaking mothers of children newly diagnosed with cancer. *Journal of Pediatric Psychology, 1*, 1–13.

Auslander, W., Haire-Joshu, D., Houston, C., Rhee, C-W., & Williams, J. (2002). A controlled evaluation of staging dietary patterns to reduce the risk of Diabetes in African American women. *Diabetes Care, 25*(5), 809–814.

Bachman, K. (2007). Obesity, weight management and health care costs: A primer. *Disease Management, 10*(3), 129–137.

Baker, A., Boggs, T., & Lewin, J. (2001). Randomized controlled trial of brief cognitive behavior intervention among regular users of amphetamine. *Addiction, 96*, 1279–1287.

Balu, S., & Thomas, J. (2006). Incremental expenditure of treating hypertension in the United States. *American Journal of Hypertension, 19*(8), 810–816.

Bean, M., Stewart, K., & Olbrisch, M. (2008). Obesity in America: Implications for clinical and health psychologists. *Journal of Clinical Psychology in Medical Settings, 15*, 214–224.

Befort, C., Nollen, N., Ellerbeck, E., Sullivan, D., Thomas, J., & Ahluwalia, J. (2008). Motivational interviewing fails to improve outcomes of a behavioral weight program for obese African American women: A pilot randomized trial. *Journal of Behavioral Medicine, 31*, 367–377.

Bertera, E. (2003). Psychosocial factors and ethnic disparities in diabetes diagnosis and treatment among older adults. *Health & Social Work, 28*(1), 33–42.

Bonner, S., Zimmerman, B., Evans, D., Trigoyen, M., Resnick, D., Mellins, R. (2002). An individualized intervention to improve asthma management among urban Latino and African American families. *Journal of Asthma, 39*(2), 167–179.

Borrelli, B., Riekert, K., Weinstein, A., & Rathier, L. (2007). Brief motivational interviewing to promote asthma medication adherence. *Journal of Allergy & Clinical Immunology, 120*, 1023–1030.

Borrelli, L. (2009). Race, ethnicity, and self-reported hypertension: Analysis of data from the National Health Interview Survey, 1997-2005. *American Journal of Public Health, 99*(2), 213–219.

Bosworth, H., Olsen, M., Neary, A., Orr, M., Grabber, J., Suvetkey, L. et al. (2008). Take control of your blood pressure (TCYB) study: A multifactorial tailored behavioral and educational intervention for achieving blood pressure control. *Patient Education & Counseling, 70*(3), 338–347.

Bradshaw, B., Richardson, G., Kumpfer, K., Carlson, J., Stanchfield, J., Overall, J. et al. (2007). Determining the efficacy of a resiliency training approach in adults with Type 2 diabetes. *The Diabetes Educator, 33*(4), 650–659.

Brown, J., Bakeman, R., Celano, M., Demi, A., Kobrynski, L., & Wilson, S. (2002). Home-based asthma education of young low-income children and their families. *Journal of Pediatric Psychology, 27*(7), 677–688.

Brown, S., Garcia, A., Kouzekanani, K., & Hanis, C. (2002). Culturally competent diabetes self-management education for Mexican Americans. *Diabetes Care, 25*, 259–268.

Brummett, B., Siegler, I., Rohe, W., Barefoot, J., Vitaliano, P., Surwit, R. et al. (2005). Neighborhood characteristics moderate effects of caregiving on glucose functioning. *Psychosomatic Medicine, 67*, 752–758.

Burgmer, R., Petersen, I., Burgmer, M., Zwaan, M., Wolf, A., & Herpertz, S. (2007). Psychological outcome two years after restrictive bariatric surgery. *Obesity Surgery, 17*, 785–791.

Burke, W. (2003). Genomics as a probe for disease biology. *New England Journal of Medicine, 349,* 969–974.

Byrne, N., Meerkin, J., Laukkanen, R., Ross, R., Fogelholm, M., & Hills, A. (2006). Weight loss strategies for obese adults: Personalized weight management vs. standard care. *Obesity, 14,* 1777–1788.

Carels, R., Darby, L., Cacciapaglia, H., Douglass, O., Harper, J., Kaplar, M. et al. (2005). Applying a stepped care approach to the treatment of obesity. *Journal of Psychosomatic Research, 59,* 375–383.

Carels, R., Darby, L., Cacciapaglia, H., Konrad, K., Coit, C., Kaplar, M. et al. (2007). Using motivational interviewing as a supplement to obesity treatment: A stepped-care approach. *Health Psychology, 26*(3), 369–374.

Carter, J., Gilliland, S., Perez, G., Levin, S., Broussard, B., Cunningham-Sabo, L. et al. (1997). Native American Diabetes Project: Designing culturally relevant education materials. *Diabetes Educator, 23,* 133–134.

Casillas, J., Zebrack, B., & Zeltzer, L. (2006). Health-related quality of life for Latino survivors of childhood cancer. *Journal of Psychosocial Oncology, 24*(3), 125–145.

Centers for Disease Control & Prevention. (2005a). *Ethnic disparities in prevalence, treatment, and control of hypertension: United States, 1999–2002. Morbidity and Mortality Weekly Report, 54,* 7–9.

Centers for Disease Control & Prevention, National Center for Health Statistics. (2005b). *National Health Interview Survey 2001–2005: Summary Health Statistics for U. S. Children.* Retrieved November 9, 2008 from www.cdc.gov/nchs/fastats/asthma.

Centers for Disease Control & Prevention. (2006a). *Chartbook on Trends in the Health of Americans.* National Center for Health Statistics. Hyattsville, MD: U.S. Department of Health and Human Services.

Centers for Disease Control & Prevention, National Center for Health Statistics. (2006b). *National Health Interview Survey, 2005: Summary Health Statistics for U. S. Children.* National Center for Health Statistics, Vital Health Statistics, *10*(231).

Centers for Disease Control & Prevention, National Center for Health Statistics. (2006c). *Prevalence of overweight and obesity among adults: United States, 2003–2004.* Retrieved September 17, 2008 from http://www.cdc.gove/nchs/products.

Chadiha, L., Proctor, E., Morrow-Howell, N., Darkwa, O., & Dore, P. (1996). Religiosity and church-based assistance among chronically ill African-American and White elderly. *Journal of Religious Gerontology, 10*(1), 17–36.

Chang, M-W., Brown, R., Baumann, L., & Nitzke, S. (2008). Self-efficacy and dietary fat reduction behaviors in obese African American and White mothers. *Obesity, 16*(5), 992–1001.

Channon, S., Huws-Thomas, M., Rollnick, S., Cannings-John, R., Rogers, C., & Gregory, J. (2007). A multicenter randomized controlled trial of motivational interviewing in teenagers with diabetes. *Diabetes Care, 30*(6), 1390–1395.

Channon, S., Smith, V., & Gregory, J. (2003). A pilot study of motivational interviewing in adolescents with diabetes. *Archives of Disease in Childhood, 88*(8), 680–683.

Choban, P., Jackson, B., Poplawski, S., & Bistolarides, P. (2002). Bariatric surgery for morbid obesity: Why, who, when, how, where, and then what? *Cleveland Clinic Journal of Medicine, 69*(11), 897–903.

Chobanian, A., Balaris, G., Black, H., Cushman, W., Green, L., Isso, D. et al. (2003). The seventh report of the joint national committee on prevention detection, evaluation, and treatment of high blood pressure. *Journal of the American Medical Association, 289*, 2560–2571.

Clark, J., & Fletcher, P. (2003). Communication issues faced by parents who have a child diagnosed with cancer. *Journal of Pediatric Oncology Nursing, 20*(4), 175–191.

Clark, N., Mitchell, H., & Rand, C. (2009). Effectiveness of educational and behavioral asthma interventions. *Pediatrics, 123*(Supplement 3 March, S185–S192).

Coffman, J., Cabana, M., Halpin, H., & Yelin, E. (2008). Effects of asthma education on children's use of acute care services: A meta-analysis. *Pediatrics, 121*, 575–586.

Colland, V. (1993). Learning to cope with asthma: A behavioural self-management program for children. *Patient Education and Counseling, 22*, 141–152.

Cornelius, D. (2000). Financial barriers to health care for Latinos: Poverty and beyond. *Journal of Poverty, 4*(1/2), 63–83.

Cox, L. (2003). A model of health behavior to guide studies of childhood cancer survivors. *Oncology Nursing Forum, 30*(5), E92–E99.

Cutler, J., Sorlie, Pl, Wolz, M., Thorn, T., Fields, L., & Roccella, E. (2008). Trends in hypertension prevalence, awareness, treatment and control rates in United States adults between 1988–1994 and 1999–2004. *Hypertension* (November), 818–227.

Davies, B., Whitsett, S., Bruce, A., & McCarthy, P. (2002). A typology of fatigue in children with cancer. *Journal of Pediatric Oncology Nursing, 19*, 12–21.

DeCoster, V. (2003). The emotions of adults with diabetes: A comparison across race. *Social Work in Health Care, 36*(4), 79–99.

DeCoster, V., & Cummings, S. (2004). Coping with Type 2 Diabetes: Do race and gender matter? *Social Work in Health Care, 40*(2), 37–53.

Dolgin, M., Somer, E., Buchvald, E., & Zaizov, R. (1999). Quality of life in adult survivors of childhood cancer. *Social Work in Health Care, 28*(4), 31–43.

Dorsten, B. (2007). The use of motivational interviewing in weight loss. *Current Diabetes Reports, 7*, 386–390.

Dreimane, D., Safani, D., MacKenzie, M., Halvorson, M., Braun, S., Conrad, B. et al. (2007). Feasibility of a hospital-based, family-centered intervention to reduce weight gain in overweight children and adolescents. *Diabetes Research and Clinical Practice, 75*, 159–168.

Drevenhorn, E., Kjellgren, K., & Bengsten, A. (2007). Outcomes following a programme for lifestyle changes with people with hypertension. *Journal of Clinical Nursing, 16*(7b), 14–151.

Egger, G. (2008). Helping patients lose weight: What works? *Australian Family Physician, 37*(1/2), 20–23.

Ellis, D., Frey, M., Naar-King, S., Templin, T., Cunningham, P., & Cakan, N. (2005). The effects of multisystemic therapy on diabetes stress among adolescents with chronically poorly controlled type 1 diabetes: Findings from a randomized, controlled trial. *Pediatrics, 116* (6), e826–832.

Emmons, K., & Rollnick, S. (2001). Motivational interviewing in health care settings. *American Journal of Preventive Medicine, 20*(1), 68–74.

Encinosa, W., Bernard, D., Steiner, C., & Chen, C-C. (2005). Use and costs of bariatric surgery and prescription weight-loss medications. *Health Affairs, 24*(4), 1039–1046.

Espinet, L., Osmick, M., Ahmend, T., & Villagra, V. (2005). A cohort study of the impact of a National Disease Management Program on HEDIS diabetes outcomes. *Disease Management, 8*(2), 86–92.

Evans, D., Clark, N., Feldman, C., Rips, J., Kaplan, D, Levison, M. et al. (1987). A school health education program for children with asthma aged 8–11 years. *Health Education Quarterly, 14*(3), 267–279.

Evans, R., Gergen, P., Mitchell, H., Kattan, M., Kercsmar, C., Crain, E. et al. (1999). A randomized clinical trial to reduce asthma morbidity among inner-city children: Results of the National Cooperative Inner-city Asthma Study. *The Journal of Pediatrics, 135*(3), 332–338.

Fitzgibbon, M., Stolley, M., Schiffer, L., Sharp, L., Singh, V., Van Horn, L. et al. (2008). Obesity reduction black intervention trial (ORBIT): Design and base-line characteristics. *Journal of Women's Health, 17*(7), 1099–1110.

Foreman, T., Willis, L., & Goodenough, B. (2005). Hospital-based support groups for parents of seriously unwell children: An example from pediatric oncology in Australia. *Social Work with Groups, 28*(2), 3–24.

Forlani, G., Zannoni, C., Tarrini, G., Melchionda, N., & Marchesini, G. (2006). An empowerment-based education program improves psychological well-being and health-related quality of life in Type 1 diabetes. *Journal of Endocrinological Investigation, 29*, 405–412.

Fox, P., Porter, P., Lob, S., Holloman, B., Rocha, D., & Adelson, J. (2007). Improving asthma-related health outcomes among low-income, multiethnic, school-aged children: Results of a demonstration project that combined continuous quality improvement and community health worker strategies. *Pediatrics, 120*, 902–911.

Friedman D., & Meadows, T. (2002). Late effects of childhood cancer therapy. *Pediatric Clinics of North America, 49*, 1083–1106.

Gallegos, E., Ovalle-Berumen, F., & Gomez-Meza, M. (2006). Metabolic control of adults with Type 2 diabetes mellitus through education and counseling. *Journal of Nursing Scholarship, 38*(4), 344–361.

Gambrill, E. (2006). Evidence-based practice and policy: Choices ahead. *Research on Social Work Practice, 16*(1), 338–357.

Gebert, N., Hummelink, R., Konnig, J., Staab, D., Schmidt, S., Szczdpanski, R. et al. (1998). Efficacy of a self-management program for childhood asthma— A prospective controlled study. *Patient Education and Counseling, 35*(3), 213–228.

Gilliland, S., Azen, S., Perez, G., & Carter, J. (2002). Strong in body and spirit: Lifestyle intervention for Native American adults with diabetes in New Mexico. *Diabetes Care, 25*(1), 78–83.

Golay, A., Lagger, G., Chambouleyron, M., Carrard, I., & Lasserre-Moutet, A. (2008). Therapeutic education of diabetic patients. *Diabetes Metabolism Research and Reviews, 24*, 192–196.

Greaves, C., Middlebrook, A., O'Loughlin, L., Holland, S., Piper, J., Steele, A. et al. (2008). Motivational interviewing for modifying diabetes risk: A randomized controlled trial. *British Journal of General Practice, 58*, 535–540.

Grey, M., Boland, E., Davidson, M., Ma, C., Sullivan-Bolyai, S., & Tamborlane, W. (1998). Short-term effects of coping skills training as adjunct to intensive therapy in adolescents. *Diabetes Care, 21*(6), 902–908.

Gross, A., Magalinck, L., & Richardson, P. (1985). Self-management training with families of insulin-dependent Diabetic children: A controlled long-term investigation. *Children and Family Behavior Therapy, 7*(1), 35–50.

Guevara, J., Wolf, F., Grum, C., & Clark, N. (2003). Effects of educational interventions for self management in children and adolescents: Systematic review and meta-analysis. *British Journal of Medicine, 26*, 1308–1314.

Halterman, J., Borrelli, B., Fisher, S., Szilagyi, P., & Yoos, L. (2008). Improving care for urban children with asthma: Design and methods of the school-based asthma therapy (SBAT) trial. *Journal of Asthma, 45*(4), 279–286.

Haynes, B., Gibbs, C., Gourash, W., Trout, S., Walters-Salas, T., Akers, R. et al. (2008). Adolescent weight loss surgery: Current issues. *Bariatric Nursing and Surgical Patient Care, 3*, 197–205.

Helmrath, M., Brandt, M., & Inge, T. (2006). Adolescent obesity and bariatric surgery. *Surgical and the Clinics of North America 86*, 441–454.

Herbert, T., & Cohen, S. (1993). Stress and immunity in humans: A meta-analytic review. *Psychosomatic Medicine, 55*, 364–379.

Hildebrandt, S. E. (1998). Effects of participation in bariatric support group after Roux-en-y gastric bypass. *Obesity Surgery, 8*, 535–542.

Hinds, P., Quargnenti, A., Bush, A., Pratt, C., Fairclough, D., Rissmiller, G. et al. (2000). An evaluation of the impact of a self-care coping intervention on psychological and clinical outcomes in adolescents with newly diagnosed cancer. *European Journal of Oncology Nursing, 18*, 6–17.

Hintsanen, M., Kivimäki, M., Elovainio, M., Pulkki-Råback, L., Keskivaara, P., Juonala, M. et al. (2005). Job strain and early atherosclerosis: The Cardiovascular Risk in Young Finns Study. *Psychosomatic Medicine, 67*, 740–747.

Hoff, A., Mullins, L., Gillaspy, S., Page, M., Pelt, J., & Chaney, J. (2005). An intervention to decrease uncertainty and distress among parents of children newly diagnosed with diabetes. *Families, Systems, & Health, 23*(3), 329–342.

Honig, P. (2005). A multi-family group programme as part of an inpatient service for adolescents with a diagnosis of anorexia nervosa. *Clinical Child Psychology and Psychiatry, 10*(4), 465–475.

Horner, S. (2004). Effect of education on school-age children's and parents' asthma management. *Journal of School Nurse Practice, 9*(3), 95–102.

Iobst, E., Alderfer, M., Olle, J., Askins, M., Fairclough, D., Katz, E. et al. (2009). Brief report: Problem solving and maternal distress at the time of a child's diagnosis of cancer in two-parent versus lone-parent households. *Journal of Pediatric Psychology 1*, 1–5.

Joseph, C., Peterson, E., Havstad, S., Johnson, C., Hoeraul, S., Stringer, S. et al. (2006). A web-based, tailored asthma management program for urban African-American high school students. *American Journal of Respiratory & Critical Care Medicine, 175*, 888–895.

Kaiser Family Foundation. (2004). *Racial and ethnic disparities in women's health coverage and access to care: Findings from the 2001 Kaiser Women's Health Survey.* Washington, DC: Author.

Kalarchian, M., Marcus, M., Levine, M., Courcoulas A., Pikonis, P., Ringham, R. et al. (2007). Psychiatric disorders among bariatric surgery candidates: Relationship to obesity and functional health status. *American Journal of Psychiatry, 164(2)*, 328–334.

Karlsen, B., Idsoe, T., Hanestad, B. Murberg. T., & Bru, K. (2004). Perceptions of support, diabetes-related coping and psychological well-being in adults with type 1 and type 2 diabetes. *Psychology, Health, & Medicine, 9(1)*, 53–70.

Katz, E., & Varni, J. (1993). Social support and social cognitive problem-solving in children with newly diagnosed cancer. *Cancer Supplement, 71(10)*, 3314–3319.

Kaugars, A., Klinnert, M., & Bender, B. (2004). Family influences on pediatric asthma. *Journal of Pediatric Psychology, 29(7)*, 475–491.

Kazak, A. (2005). Evidence-based interventions for survivors of childhood cancer and their families. *Journal of Pediatric Psychology, 30(1)*, 29–39.

Kazak, A., & Baxt, C. (2007). Families of infants and young children with cancer: A post-traumatic stress framework. *Pediatric Blood Cancer, 49*, 1109–1113.

Kazak, A., Alderfer, M., Streisand, R., Simms, S., Rourke, M., Barakat, L. et al. (2004). Treatment of posttraumatic stress symptoms in adolescent survivors of childhood cancer and their families: A randomized clinical trial. *Journal of Family Psychology, 18(3)*, 493–504.

Kazak, A., Barak, L., Meeske, K., Christakis, D., Meadows, A., Casey, R. et al. (1997). Posttraumatic stress, family functioning, and social support of survivors of childhood leukemia and their mothers and fathers. *Journal of Consulting and Clinical Psychology, 65*, 120–129.

Kazak, A., Simms, S., Alderfer, M., Rourke, M., Crump, T., McClure, K. et al. (2005). Feasability and preliminary outcomes from a pilot study of a brief psychological intervention for families of children newly diagnosed with cancer. *Journal of Pediatric Psychology, 30(8)*, 655–655.

Kazak, A., Simms, S., Barakat, L., Hobbie, W., Foley, B. Golomb, V. et al. (1999). Surviving Cancer Competently Intervention Program (SCCIP): A cognitive-behavioral and family therapy intervention for adolescent survivors of childhood cancer and their families. *Family Process, 38*, 175–191.

Kivirmäki, M., Ferrie, J., Brunner, F., Head, J., Shipley, M., Vahtera, J. et al. (2005). Justice at work and reduced risk of coronary heart disease among employees: The Whitehall II Study. *Archives of Internal Medicine, 165*, 2245–2251.

Klinnert, M., Kaugars, A., Strand, M., & Veira, L. (2008). Family psychological factors in relation to children's asthma status and behavioral adjustment at age 4. *Family Process, 47*, 41–61.

Klosky, J., Garces-Webb, D., Buscemi, J., Schum, L., Tyc, V., & Merchant, T. (2007). Examination of an interactive-educational intervention in improving parent and child distress in radiation procedures. *Children's Healthcare, 36(4)*, 323–334.

Klosky, J., Tyc, V., Srivastava, D., Tong, K., Kronenberg, M., Booker, Z. et al. (2004). Brief report: Evaluation of an interactive intervention designed to reduce pediatric distress during radiation therapy procedures. *Journal of Pediatric Psychology, 29(8)*, 621–626.

Knight, K., McGowan, L., Dickens, C., & Bundy, C. (2006). A systematic review of motivational interviewing in physical health settings. *British Journal of Health Psychology, 11*, 319–332.

Koocher, G., & O'Malley, J. (1981). *The Damocles syndrome: Psychological consequences of surviving childhood cancer*. NewYork: McGraw-Hill.

Krishna, S., Balas, E., Francisco, B., & Konig, P. (2006). Effective and sustainable multimedia education for children with asthma: A randomized controlled trial. *Children's Healthcare, 35*(1), 75–90.

Lang, A., & Froelicher, E. (2006). Management of overweight and obesity in adults: Behavioral interventions for long-term weight loss and maintenance. *European Journal of Cardiovascular Nursing, 5*, 102–114.

Lara, M., Rosenbaum, S., Rachelefsky, G., Nicholas, W., Morton, S., Emont, S. et al. (2002). Improving childhood asthma outcomes in the United States: A blueprint for policy action. *Pediatrics, 109*(5), 919–929.

LaRoche, M., Koinis-Mitchell, D., & Gualdron, L. (2006). A culturally competent asthma management intervention: A randomized controlled pilot study. *Annals of Allergy, Asthma & Immunology, 96* (January), 80–85.

Latner, J., Wilson, G., Stunkard, A., & Jackson, M. (2002). Self-help and long-term behavior therapy for obesity. *Behavior Research and Therapy, 40*, 805–812.

LaViest, T. (1993). Segregation, poverty, and empowerment: Health consequences for African Americans. *Millbank Quarterly, 71*, 41–64.

Lee, J., Parker, V., & DuBose, L. (2008). Demands and resources: Parents of school-age children with asthma. *Journal of Pediatric Nursing, 21*(9), 425–433.

Lemmens, G., Eisler, I., Migerode, L., Heireman, M., & Demyttenaere, K. (2007). Family discussion group therapy for major depression: A brief systemic multi-family group intervention for hospitalized patients and their family members. *Journal of Family Therapy, 29*(1), 49–68.

Lesley, M. (2007). Social problem solving training for African Americans: Effects on dietary problem solving skill and DASH diet-related behavior change. *Patient Education and Counseling, 65*, 137–146.

Levine, M., Ringham, R., Kalarchian, M., Wisniewski, L., & Marcus, M. (2001). Is family-based behavioral weight control appropriate for severe pediatric obesity? *International Journal of Eating Disorders, 30*, 318–328.

Levy, M., Heffner, B., Stewart, T., & Beeman, G. (2006). The efficacy of asthma case management in an urban school district in reducing school absences and hospitalizations for asthma. *Journal of School Health, 76*(6), 320–324.

Lieu, P., Lozano, J., Finkelstein, F., Chi, N., Jensvold, N., Capra, A. et al. (2002). Racial/ethnic variations in asthma status and management practices among children in managed Medicaid. *Pediatrics, 109*, 857–865.

Linden, W., & Moseley, J. (2006). The efficacy of behavioral treatments for hypertension. *Applied Psychophysiology and Biofeedback, 31*(1), 51–63.

Littrell, J. (2008). New developments in understanding cardiovascular disease and the implications for social work. *Social work in Healthcare, 46*(2), 35–49.

Lorig, K., Ritter, P., & Jacquez, A. (2005). Outcomes of border health Spanish/English chronic disease self-management programs. *Diabetes Educator, 31*(3), 401–409.

Mailick, M., Holden, G., & Walther, V. (1994). Coping with childhood asthma: Caretakers' views. *Health & Social Work, 19*(2), 103–111.

Marsac, J., Funk, J., & Nelson, L. (2006). Coping styles, psychological functioning and quality of life in children with asthma. *Child Care, Health and Development, 33*(4), 360–267.

McCarthy, M., Herbert, R., Brimacombe, M., Hansen, J., Wong, D., & Zehman, M. (2002). Empowering parents through asthma education. *Pediatric Nursing, 28*(5), 464–473.

McCraty, R., Atkinson, M., & Tomasino, D. (2003). Impact of a workplace stress reduction program on blood pressure and emotional health in hypertensive employees. *Journal of Alternative and Complementary Medicine, 9*(3), 355–369.

McCunney, R. (2005). Asthma, genes, and air pollution. *Journal of Environmental Medicine, 47*(12), 1285–1291.

McGhan, S., Wong, E., Jhangri, G., Wells, Michaelchuk, M., Boechler, V. et al. (2003). Evaluation of an education program for elementary school children with asthma. *Journal of Asthma, 40*(5), 523–533.

McHugh, F., Lindsay, G., Hanlon, P., Hutton, I., Brown, M., Morrison, C. et al. (2001). Nurse led shared care for patients on the waiting list for coronary artery bypass surgery: A randomized controlled trial. *Heart, 86*, 317–323.

McNabb, W., Quinn, M., Murphy, D., Thorp, F., & Cook, S. (1995). Increasing children's responsibility for diabetes self-care: The *In Control* Study. *Diabetes Educator, 18*(7), 121–124.

McNeill, T. (2006). Evidence-based practice in an age of relativism: Toward a model of practice. *Social Work, 51*(2), 147–156.

McPherson, A., Glazebrook, C., Forster, D., James, C., & Smith, A. (2006). A randomized, controlled trial of an interaction educational compueter package for children with asthma. *Pediatrics, 117*(4), 1046–1054.

McQuaid, E., Kopel, S., & Nassau, J. (2000). Behavioral adjustment in children with asthma: A meta-analysis. *Journal of Developmental Behavioral Pediatrics, 22*, 430–490.

McQuaid, E. L., & Nassau, J. H. (1999). Empirically supported treatments in pediatric psychology: Asthma, diabetes, and cancer. *Journal of Pediatric Psychology, 24*, 305–328.

Melcher, J., & Bostwick, G. (1998). The obese client: Myths, facts, assessment, and intervention. *Health & Social Work, 23*(3), 195–202.

Morisky, D., Lees, M., Sharif, B. A., Liu, K., & Ward, H. (2002). Reducing disparities in hypertension control: A community-based hypertension control project (CHIP) for an ethnically diverse population. *Health Promotion Practice, 3*(2), 264–275.

Mullen, E., Bledsoe, S., & Bellamy, J. (2008). Implementing evidence-based social work practice. *Research on Social Work Practice, 18*(4), 325–338.

National Cancer Institute (NCI). (2006a) Cancer epidemiology in older adolescents and young adults 15–29 years of age, 1975–2000. Retrieved December 10, 2008 from www.seer_cancer.gov/publications/aya.

National Cancer Institute (NCI). (2006b). SEER Cancer Statistics Review, 1975–2003. Retrieved December 10, 2008 from www.seer_cancer.gov/csr/1975–2003.

National Center for Health Statistics. (2006). *Health, United States: With chartbook on trends in the health of Americans.* Hyattsville, MD: National Center for Health Statistics.

National Diabetes Information Clearinghouse (NDIC). (2005). *National Diabetes Fact Sheet.* National Institute of Diabetes and Digestive and Kidney Diseases, U.S. Department of Health and Human Services, National Institutes of Health. Retrieved January 15, 2009 from http://diabetes.niddk.nih.gov/dm/pubs/statistics/#7.

National Institutes of Health. (2000). *Practical guide to the identification, evaluation, and treatment of overweight and obesity in adults.* Bethesda, MD: National Institutes of Health.

Ng, S., Li, A., Lou, V., Tso, I., Wan, P., & Chan, T. (2008). Incorporating family therapy into asthma group intervention: A randomized waitlist controlled trial. *Family Process, 47*(1), 115–130.

Nguyen, N., Root, J., Zainabadi, K., Sabio, A., Chalifoux, S., Stevens, M. et al. (2005). Accelerated growth of bariatric surgery with the introduction of minimally invasive surgery. *Archives of Surgery, 140*(12), 1198–1202.

Nickel, C., Tanca, S., Kolowos, S., Pedrosa-Gil, F., & Bachler, E. (2007). Men with chronic occupational stress benefit from behavioral/psychoeducational group training: A randomized, prospective, controlled trial. *Psychological Medicine, 37*(1), 1141–1149.

Ogden, C., Carroll, M., Curtin, L., McDowell, M., Tabak, C., & Flegal, K. (2006). Prevalence of overweight and obesity in the United States, 1999–2004. *Journal of the American Medical Association, 295*(213), 1549–1555.

Ogden, C., Flegal, K., Carroll, C., & Johnson, L. (2002). Prevalence and trends in overweight among US children and adolescents. *JAMA, 288,* 1728–1732.

Onnis, L., DiGennaro, A., Cespa, G., Dentale, R., Benedetti, P., Forato, F. et al. (2001). Prevention of chronicity in psychosomatic illness: A systemic research study into the treatment of childhood asthma. *Families, Systems, & Health, 19*(3), 237–250.

Painot, D., Jotterand, S., Kammer, A., Fossati, M., & Golay, A. (2001). Simultaneous nutritional cognitive-behavioural therapy in obese patients. *Patient Education and Counseling, 42,* 47–52.

Parker-Oliver, D. (2005). Asthma management: A role for social work. *Health & Social Work, 30*(2), 167–171.

Patenaude, A., & Kupst, M. (2005). Psychosocial functioning in pediatric cancer. *Journal of Pediatric Psychology, 30*(1), 9–27.

Perri, M., Nezu, A., McKelvey, W., Shermer, R, Renjilian, D., & Viegener, B. (2001). Relapse prevention training and problem-solving therapy in the long-term management of obesity. *Journal of Consulting and Clinical Psychology, 69*(4), 722–726.

Perrin, J., Maclean, W., Gortmaker, S., & Asher, K. (1992). Improving the psychological status of children with asthma: A randomized controlled trial. *Journal of Developmental and Behavioral Pediatrics, 13*(4), 241–247.

Philis-Tsimikas, A., & Walker, C. (2001). Improved care for diabetes in underserved populations. *Journal of Ambulatory Care, 24*(1), 39–43.

Pinquart, M., & Sorensen, S. (2005). Ethnic differences in stressors, resources, and psychological outcomes of family caregiving: A meta-analysis. *The Gerontologist, 45,* 90–106.

Pulcini, J., DeSisto, M., & McIntyre, C. (2007). An intervention to increase the use of asthma action plans in schools: A MASNRN study. *The Journal of School Nursing, 23*(3), 170–176.

Quin, S. (2004). The long-term psychosocial effects of cancer diagnosis and treatment on children and their families. *Social Work in Health Care, 39*(12), 129–149.

Resnicow, K. Jackson, A., Wang, T., De, A., McCarty, F., Dudley, W. et al. (2001). A motivational interviewing intervention to increase fruit and vegetable intake through Black churches: Results of the *Eat for Life Trial. American Journal of Public Health, 91*, 1686–1693.

Rich-Edwards, J., & Grizzard, T. (2005). Psychosocial stress and neuroendoctrine mechanisms in preterm delivery. *American Journal of Obstetrics and Gynecology, 192*, S30–35.

Rubak, S., Sandboek, A., Lauritzen, T., & Christensen, B. (2005). Motivational interviewing: A systematic review and meta-analysis. *British Journal of General Practice*, April, 305–312.

Sacks, F., Svetkey, L., Vollmer, W., Appel, L., Bray, G., Harsha, D. et al. (2001). Effects on blood pressure of reduced dietary sodium and the Dietary Approaches to Stop Hypertension (DASH) DASH-Sodium. *New England Journal of Medicine, 344*, 3–10.

Sahler, J., Fairclough, D., Phipps, S., Mulhelm, R., Dolgin, M., Noll, R. et al. (2005). Using problem-solving skills training to reduce negative affectivity in mothers of children with newly diagnosed cancer: Report of a multisided randomized trial. *Journal of Consulting and Clinical Psychology, 73*(2), 272–283.

Sahler, J., Varni, J., Fairclough, D., Butler, R., Noll, R. B., Dolgin, M. et al. (2002). Problem-solving skills training for mothers of children with newly diagnosed cancer: A randomized trial. *Journal of Developmental & Behavioral Pediatrics, 23*, 77–86.

Sales, J., Fivush, R., & Teague, G. (2008). The role of parental coping in children with asthma's psychological well-being and asthma-related quality of life. *Journal of Pediatric Psychology, 33*(2), 208–219.

Santry, H., Gillen, D., & Lauderdale, D. (2005). Trends in bariatric surgical procedures. *Journal of the American Medical Association, 294*(15), 1904–1917.

Sawyer, M., Spurrier, N., Whaites, L., Kennedy, D., Martin, A., & Baghurst, P. (2001). The relationship between asthma severity, family functioning and the health-related quality of life of children with asthma. *Quality of Life Research, 9*, 1105–1115.

Scarr, S. (1998). How people make their own environments: Implications for parents and policy makers. *Psychology, Public Policy and Law, 2*(2), 204–228.

Schmaling, K., Blume, A., & Afari, N. (2001). A randomized controlled pilot study of motivational interviewing to change attitudes about adherence to medications for asthma. *Journal of Clinical Psychology in Medical Settings, 8*(3), 167–172.

Schwartz, C. (2003). Health status of childhood cancer survivors: Cure is more than the eradication of cancer. *Journal of the American Medical Association, 290*(12), 1641–1643.

Shaw, S., Marshak, H., Dyjack, D., & Neish. B. (2005). Effects of a classroom-based asthma education curriculum on asthma knowledge, attitudes, self-efficacy, quality of life, and self-management behaviors among adolescents. *American Journal of Health Education, 38*(3), 140–145.

Shegog, R., Bartholomew, K., Parcel, G., Sockrider, M., Masse, L., & Abramson, S. (2001). Impact of a computer-assisted education program on factors related to asthma self-management behavior. *Journal of the American Medical Informatics Association, 8*(1), 49–61.

Smith, D., Heckemeyer, C., Kratt, P., & Mason, D. (1997). Motivational interviewing to improve adherence to a behavioral weight-control program for older women with NIDDM: A pilot study. *Diabetes Care, 20*, 52–58.

Smith-West, D., DiLillo, V., Bursac, Z., Gore, S, & Greene, P. (2007). Motivational interviewing improves weight loss in women with Type 2 diabetes. *Diabetes Care, 30*(5), 1081–1087.

Sogg, S., & Gorman, M. (2008). Interpersonal changes and challenges after weight-loss surgery. *Primary Psychiatry, 15*(8), 61–66.

Stern, M., Gonzalez, C., Mitchell, B., Villalpando, E., Haffner, S., & Hazuda, H. (1992). Genetic and environmental determinants of type II diabetes in Mexico City and San Antonio. *Diabetes, 41*, 484–492.

Stewart, A., & Davis, K. (2003). Effect of telephonic intervention on the adherence of patients with hypertension. *South African Journal of Physiotherapy, 59*(1), 29–35.

Stotts, A., Schmitz, J., Rhoades, H., & Grabowski, J. (2001). Motivational interviewing with cocaine-dependent patients: A pilot study. *Journal of Consulting Clinical Psychology, 69*, 858–862.

Sudha, S., & Multran, E. (2001). Race and ethnicity, nativity, and issues of health care. *Research on Aging, 23*(1), 3–13.

Svavarsdottir, E., McCubbin, M., & Kane, J. (2000). Well-being of parents of young children with asthma. *Research in Nursing & Health, 23*, 346–358.

Tal, D., Gil-Spielberg, S., Antonovsky, H., Tal, A., Moaz, B. (1990). Teaching families to cope with childhood asthma. *Family Systems Medicine, 8*(2), 135–144.

Thompson, S., Auslander, W., & White, N. (2001). Influence of family structure on health among youths with diabetes. *Health & Social Work, 26*(1), 7–14.

Toelle, B., Peat, J., Salome, C., Mellis, C., Bauman, A., & Woolcock, A. (1993). Evaluation of a community-based asthma management program in a population sample of school children. *The Medical Journal of Australia, 158*(7), 742–746.

Tonstad, S., Søderblom, C. & Sandvik, E. (2007). Effect of nurse counseling on metabolic risk factors in patients with mild hypertension: A randomized controlled trial. *European Journal of Cardiovascular Nursing, 6*, 160–164.

Tsai, A., Inge, T., & Burd, R. (2007). Bariatric surgery in adolescents: Recent national trends in use and in-hospital outcome. *Archives of Pediatric Adolescent Medicine, 161*, 217–221.

Tsai, A., & Wadden, T. (2005). Systematic review: An evaluation of major commercial weight loss programs in the United States. *Annals of Internal Medicine, 142*, 56–66.

Tsai, A., Wadden, T., Pillitteri, J., Sembower, M., Gerlach, K., Kyle, T. et al. (2009). Disparities of ethnicities and socioeconomic status in use of weight loss treatments. *Journal of the National Medical Association, 101*(1), 62–70.

Vallis, T., Butler, G., Perey, B., van Zanten, S., MacDonald, A., Konok, G. et al. (2001). The role of psychological functioning in morbid obesity and its treatment with gastroplasty. *Obesity surgery*, *11*, 717–725.

van Hout, G., Boekestein, P., Fortuin, F., Pelle, A., & van Heck, G. (2006). Psychosocial functioning following bariatric surgery. *Obesity Surgery*, *16*, 787–794.

van Hout, G., Fortuin, F., Pelle, A., & Guus, L. (2008). Psychosocial functioning, personality, and body image following vertical banded gastroplasty. *Obesity Surgery*, *18*, 115–120.

Varni, J., Katz, E., Colegrove, R., & Dolgin, M. (1993). The impact of social skills training on the adjustment of children with newly diagnosed cancer. *Journal of Pediatric Psychology*, *18*(6), 751–766.

Varni, J., Sahler, J., Katz, E., Mulhern, R., Copeland, D., Noll, R. et al. (1999). Maternal problem-solving therapy in pediatric cancer. *Journal of Psychosocial Oncology*, *16*, 41–71.

Velsor-Friedrich, B., Pigott, T., & Louloudes, A. (2004). The effects of a school-based intervention on the self-care and health of African American inner-city children with asthma. *Journal of Pediatric Nursing*, *19*(4), 247–256.

Vincent, D., Pasvogel, A., & Barrera, L. (2007). A feasibility study of a culturally tailored diabetes intervention for Mexican Americans. *Biological Research Nursing*, *9*(2), 130–141.

Viner, R., Christie, D., Taylor, V., & Hey, S. (2003). Motivational/solution-focused intervention improves HbA1c in adolescents with Type 1 diabetes: A pilot study. *Diabetic Medicine*, *20*, 739–742.

Wadden, T., Sarwer, D., Fabricatore, A., Jones, L., Stack, R., & Williams, N. (2007). Psychosocial and behavioral status of patients undergoing bariatric surgery: What to expect before and after surgery. *Medical Clinics in North America*, *91*, 451–469.

Wade, S. (2000). Psychosocial components of asthma management in children. *Disease Management & Health Outcomes*, *8*(1), 17–27.

Walders, N., Keresma, C., Schluchter, M., Redline, S., Kirchner, H., & Drotar, D. (2006). An interdisciplinary intervention for undertreated pediatric asthma. *CHEST*, *129*, 292–299.

Wamboldt, M., & Levin, L. (1995). Utility of multifamily psychoeducation groups for medically ill children and adolescents. *Family Systems Medicine*, *13*(2), 151–161.

Warschburger, P., von Scherin, A-D, Burchholz, H., & Petermann, F. (2002). An educational program for parents of asthmatic preschool children: Short- and medium-term effects. *Patient Education and Counseling*, *51*, 83–91.

Weil, M., Wade, S., Bauman, L., Lynn, H., Mitchell, & Lavigne, J. (1999). The relationship between psychosocial factors and asthma morbidity in inner-city children with asthma. *Pediatrics*, *104*(6), 1274–1280.

Weiner, L., Battles, H., Bernstein, D., Long, L., Derdak, J., Mackall, C. et al. (2006). Persistent psychological distress in long-term survivors of pediatric sarcoma: The experience at a single institution. *Psychological Oncology*, *15*(10), 898–910.

Welch, G., Wesolowski, C., Piepul, B., Kuhn, J., Romanelli, J., & Garb. J. (2008). Physical activity predicts weight loss following gastric bypass surgery: Findings from a support group survey. *Obesity Surgery*, *18*, 517–524.

Whitsett, S., Gudmundsdottir, M., Davies, B., McCarthy, P., & Friedman, D. (2008). Chemotherapy-related fatigue in childhood cancer: Correlates, consequences, and coping strategies. *Children's Healthcare, 36*(4), 323–334.

Wood, B., Lim, J., Miller, B., Cheah, P., Ann, P., Simmens, S. et al. (2007). Family emotional climate, depression, emotional triggering of asthma, and disease severity in pediatric asthma: Examination of pathways of effect. *Journal of Pediatric Psychology, 32*(5), 542–551.

Wyatt, S., Akylbekova, E., Wofford, M., Coady, S., Walker, E., Andrew, M. et al. (2008). Prevalence, awareness, treatment, and control of hypertension in the Jackson Heart Study. *Hypertension, 51,* 650–656.

Wysocki, T., Harris, M. A., Buckloh, L., Mertlich, D., Lochrie, A., Mauras, N. et al. (2007). Randomized trial of behavioral family systems therapy for Diabetes. *Diabetes Care, 30*(3), 555–560.

Wysocki, T., Harris, M., Greco, P., Bubb, J., Danda, C., Harvey, L. et al. (2000). Randomized, controlled trial of behavior therapy for families of adolescents with insulin dependent diabetes mellitus. *Journal of Pediatric Psychology, 25*(1), 23–33.

Yin, T., Wu, F-L., Liu, Y-L., & Yu, S. (2005). Effects of weight-loss program for obese children: A "mix of attributes" approach. *Journal of Nursing Research, 13,* 21–29.

Yorke, J., & Shuldman, C. (2009). *Family therapy for asthma in children.* The Cochrane Collaboration. Retrieved January 31, 2009 from http://www.thecochranelibrary.com.

Zebrack, B., & Chesler, M. (2002). Quality of life in childhood cancer survivors. *Psycho-Oncology, 11,* 132–141.

Zebrack, B., Chesler, M., Orbuch, T., & Parry, C. (2002). Mothers of survivors of childhood cancer: Their worries and concerns. *Journal of Psychosocial Oncology, 20*(2), 1–25.

Zebrack, B., Gurney, J., Oeffinger, K., Whitton, J., Packer, R., Mertens, A. et al. (2004). Psychological outcomes in long-term survivors of childhood brain cancer: A report from the Childhood Cancer Survivor Study. *Journal of Clinical Oncology, 22,* 999–1006.

Zebrack, B., Zeltzer, L., Whitton, J., Mertens, A., Odom, L., Berkow, R. et al. (2002). Psychological outcomes in long-term survivors of childhood leukemia, Hodgkin's disease, and non-Hodgkin's lymphoma: A report from the Childhood Cancer Survivor Study. *Pediatrics, 110,* 42–52.

Zhu, Y., Stovall, J., Buter, L., Ji, Q., Gaber, M., & Samant, S. (2000). Comparison of two immobilization techniques using portal film and digitally reconstructed radiographs for pediatric patients with brain tumors. *International Journal of Radiation Oncology, Biology, Physics, 48,* 1233–1240.

Zlotnick, J., & Galambos, C. (2004). Evidence-based practices in health care: Social work responsibilities. *Health & Social Work, 29*(4), 259–261.

Index

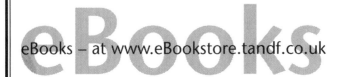